## Praise for *The Tapping Solution for Weight Loss and Body Confidence*

"As a physician fully aware of the many health benefits of maintaining a healthy weight, I've long been on the lookout for a book I could recommend to patients who were ready to get off the dieting treadmill and really do the internal work necessary in order to achieve an optimally healthy weight *permanently.* Look no further. This is that book."

— LISSA RANKIN, M.D., OB/GYN, *New York Times* best-selling author of *Mind Over Medicine*

"*Change your plate, change your fate* has been one of my favorite mottos for years. But sadly, it's difficult to nourish our bodies when our self-worth is in the toilet. *The Tapping Solution for Weight Loss and Body Confidence* is a powerful system that releases the emotions and beliefs that hold us back from loving our bodies. I use tapping on a regular basis and have personally benefited from this powerful method. It's one of the most important practices in my healing arsenal. Join Jessica Ortner on this amazing journey and give it a try!"

— KRIS CARR, *New York Times* best-selling author of *Crazy Sexy Kitchen*

"I'm so excited about this book! Tapping is a powerful tool that allows people to make positive changes in record time, and I'm thrilled that Jessica Ortner has brought this life-changing technique to women who long to feel good in their bodies. By dealing with the source of the problem—the pain beneath your weight, the beliefs that keep you stuck, or the boundaries that need to be set—you won't have to wait to lose weight to feel confident. You can feel good *right now* by simply doing the exercises in this book. *The Tapping Solution for Weight Loss and Body Confidence* may just go down in history as a game-changer when it comes to leading women out of weight loss hell."

— CHERYL RICHARDSON, *New York Times*
**best-selling author of *The Art of Extreme Self-Care***


"This book is awesome! I was hooked on the first page. Jessica empowers you by showing you how to *energetically* remove the obstacles. I love it; it is such a fun read, so personal, and I recommend it highly to everyone who has struggled with their weight. Thank you, Jessica Ortner, for writing a beautiful book that will help people succeed . . . easily."

— DONNA EDEN, **author of *Energy Medicine***
**and *Energy Medicine for Women***


"Jessica Ortner not only gently teaches tools to change lives now, she also inspires us to embrace our uniqueness and to love ourselves completely. If only every teenage girl in America could be taught this type of self-love and body confidence . . ."

— DONNA GATES, **author of *The Body Ecology Diet***

"In *The Tapping Solution for Weight Loss and Body Confidence*, Jessica Ortner offers an effective, practical approach to eliminating self-judgment and criticism toward our bodies. If we want deep and lasting change in our weight and our confidence, we have to let go of the negative beliefs and emotions that hold us back. Tapping is one of the most powerful techniques I've experienced to do that, and Jessica is the perfect guide on the journey toward greater self-love and confidence."

— MARCI SHIMOFF, #1 *New York Times* best-selling author of *Happy for No Reason, Love for No Reason*, and *Chicken Soup for the Woman's Soul*

"*The Tapping Solution for Weight Loss and Body Confidence* is a must read! Jessica Ortner brilliantly empowers readers to face their fears to establish a new relationship to their body. Her EFT expertise shines through each page of the book as she simplifies the technique for the newcomer while greatly supporting those who have been on a lifelong path. I love this book!"

— GABRIELLE BERNSTEIN, *New York Times* best-selling author of *May Cause Miracles*

"*The Tapping Solution for Weight Loss and Body Confidence* is an empowering and effective guide to quickly and painlessly becoming the person you know yourself to authentically be in the body you want to have. Using this guide will ease you into your best self in every way, once and for all. Get it, use it, and enjoy now and forever the freedom it brings."

— SONIA CHOQUETTE, *New York Times* best-selling author of *The Answer Is Simple*

"Jessica's book, *The Tapping Solution for Weight Loss and Body Confidence,* is full of compassion and provides a key that can unlock fat storage. Success is available with tapping by eliminating your negative self-talk and opening up the opportunity to cherish your personal beauty."

—JULIE DANILUK, **author of *Meals that Heal Inflammation***

"A strong beautiful body comes from quieting all the noise and stress about diet and exercise so that we can hear and follow our own intuition. Using tapping, Jessica teaches us how to do just that and radiate from the inside out. Let go of the stress and begin to thrive."

—TARA STILES, **founder of Strala and author of *Slim Calm Sexy Yoga***

"This is no ordinary weight loss book. This is a road map, memoir, and instruction manual for a life well lived in a body well loved. I love Jessica Ortner's combination of vulnerability, humor, and tested tapping scripts. Reading this gave me new insight into how mind and body can be yoked together to work as a supportive team to create a vibrant body and life."

—ALEXANDRA JAMIESON, **co-creator of *Super Size Me* and author of *The Great American Detox Diet***

"Who would have thought that a book about *weight loss* could feel like a warm hug and a cup of steaming hot cocoa with a great friend? That is the brilliance of Jessica Ortner. She accompanies us deep inside our core issues, with amazing compassion and incredible tools and technology that produce outstanding results. I recommend this book to anyone who has always wanted to find her way home to the body she was born to love."

—REGENA THOMASHAUER, **author of *Mama Gena's School of Womanly Arts***

"If you're ready to embody your true power and melt away your struggle with weight, Jessica has the solution. Read this now. Because you deserve to feel as beautiful as you truly are."

— MARIE FORLEO, **author of** *Make Every Man Want You*

"In a culture obsessed with quick fixes, fad diets, and the circumference of a supermodel's thighs, Jessica Ortner's book stands out as an empowering solution to the weight-watching woes of the modern woman. Jessica addresses the fear, tension, and pain that keep women looped in a cycle of self-destructive habits, offering tools for self-reflection, healing, and personal growth. Using the renowned EFT method, Jessica offers a solution that addresses your spirit, mind, *and* waistline. This book will help you pick up the pieces and reclaim your body as sacred, sexy, and beautiful."

— LATHAM THOMAS, **author of** *Mama Glow*

"Jessica Ortner really has her finger on the pulse when it comes to stress-related weight gain and how to avoid the effects of stress on the body. Tapping is a great solution to break the stress response and restore the body to its proper metabolic function. I love how Jessica makes it safe to be honest about our real, sometimes unconscious, eating habits by being so open and aware of her own issues. She is an inspiration and has a solution-oriented approach to an issue that plagues many women and is ultimately linked to our overall confidence. You go girl!"

— LISA GARR, **host of** *The Aware Show*

"In *The Tapping Solution for Weight Loss and Body Confidence,* Jessica Ortner has provided a tremendous resource, for not only women but also teenage girls to help them release the shame and bondage so commonly associated with weight and appearance. As an expert in women's issues, I applaud her for creating such a valuable and timely resource to help free women from these false beliefs and misperceptions about themselves. Any woman who reads this book will be set free to feel more love and appreciation for herself and more joy in all areas of life."

— CAROL TUTTLE, **creator of dressingyourtruth.com**

"Jessica's book is a treasure! It's filled with tools, strategies, and insights on how to get you to a more loving and accepting place for yourself and to release the real issues behind weight gain. You will feel like you're hearing from a loving, kind best friend. I continuously experience the difference tapping makes in my own life and the relief it provides. If you want to feel a shift, read and practice what's in this book."

— AGAPI STASSINOPOULOS, **author of** *Unbinding the Heart*

"Jessica Ortner reminds us that there's nothing more important than healing our relationship with our own body. Somehow we've forgotten the sacred gift it is—the fact that it's our chance to be here. With humor and humility, Jessica reveals a very simple tool that radically shifts our experience of being embodied from self-hatred to self-acceptance. At the very least, you'll find more wellness by reading this book. At most, you'll transform your entire life."

— MEGGAN WATTERSON, **author of** *Reveal*

"As a fitness expert, people ask me all the time what exercise they should do and what food they should eat to lose weight. The answer is never simple, because it goes so much deeper than just exercise and diet. Jessica beautifully goes where many weight loss books are unwilling to go, diving gracefully into the underlying emotional and physiological blocks that keep women from making big changes in their bodies and lives. She offers *profound* yet *simple* exercises that *will* work fast. Having tapped with her, I know firsthand that her work is filled with love, wisdom, and genuine compassion—she's simply magical, as is this book."

— ERIN STUTLAND, **creator of Shrink Session Workout**

"In *The Tapping Solution for Weight Loss and Body Confidence,* Jessica Ortner gives readers a way to embrace self-love and acceptance and cut through all of the limiting habits and beliefs that contribute to being overweight. While tapping may seem too simple or strange, it absolutely works. Jessica is going to help millions of people love themselves to their ideal bodies and, even better, their ideal lives."

— HEATHER DANE, **health coach**

"EFT is a simple, time-friendly, miracle-producing tool that immediately transmutes and transforms limiting thoughts, beliefs and even physical ailments. *The Tapping Solution for Weight Loss and Body Confidence* delivers profound insights and proven processes for achieving life-changing mental and physical balance and restoring overall vitality."

—JENNIFER McLEAN, **author, healer, and host of** *Healing with the Masters*

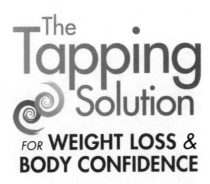

The Tapping Solution for WEIGHT LOSS & BODY CONFIDENCE

# The Tapping Solution

## FOR WEIGHT LOSS & BODY CONFIDENCE

A Woman's Guide *to* Stressing Less,
Weighing Less *and* Loving More

JESSICA ORTNER

**HAY HOUSE**

Carlsbad, California • New York City • London • Sydney
Johannesburg • Vancouver • Hong Kong • New Delhi

**First published and distributed in the United Kingdom by:**
Hay House UK Ltd, Astley House, 33 Notting Hill Gate, London W11 3JQ
Tel: +44 (0)20 3675 2450; Fax: +44 (0)20 3675 2451
www.hayhouse.co.uk

**Published and distributed in the United States of America by:**
Hay House Inc., PO Box 5100, Carlsbad, CA 92018-5100
Tel: (1) 760 431 7695 or (800) 654 5126
Fax: (1) 760 431 6948 or (800) 650 5115
www.hayhouse.com

**Published and distributed in Australia by:**
Hay House Australia Ltd, 18/36 Ralph St, Alexandria NSW 2015
Tel: (61) 2 9669 4299; Fax: (61) 2 9669 4144
www.hayhouse.com.au

**Published and distributed in the Republic of South Africa by:**
Hay House SA (Pty) Ltd, PO Box 990, Witkoppen 2068
Tel/Fax: (27) 11 467 8904
www.hayhouse.co.za

**Published and distributed in India by:**
Hay House Publishers India, Muskaan Complex, Plot No.3, B-2,
Vasant Kunj, New Delhi 110 070
Tel: (91) 11 4176 1620; Fax: (91) 11 4176 1630
www.hayhouse.co.in

**Distributed in Canada by:**
Raincoast Books, 2440 Viking Way, Richmond, B.C. V6V 1N2
Tel: (1) 604 448 7100; Fax: (1) 604 270 7161; www.raincoast.com

The information given in this book should not be treated as a substitute for professional
medical advice; always consult a medical practitioner. Any use of information in this book
is at the reader's discretion and risk. Neither the author nor the publisher can be held responsible for any loss, claim or damage arising out of the use, or misuse, of the suggestions
made, the failure to take medical advice or for any material on third party websites.

A catalogue record for this book is available from the British Library.

ISBN: 978-1-78180-291-5

Printed and bound in Great Britain by TJ International, Padstow, Cornwall.

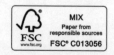

To the women who have so generously shared
their stories with me and encouraged me to share mine.

We shine brighter together.

# Contents

# Foreword

This book came into my life at exactly the right time . . . about a month before a photo shoot for the cover of my latest book. I've been doing photo shoots for years, and leading up to each shoot, I would be concerned about fitting into the right size clothing. Then I'd immediately put myself on a strict diet so that my clothes would fit on the day of the shoot. For weeks beforehand, I would cut my calories and weigh myself daily. I would even travel with my scale. And this worked for years. Until it stopped working. That's right. My body finally said "No more." No amount of caloric restriction or exercise worked anymore. The scale—and my size—simply wouldn't budge. I know this flies in the face of how biology is supposed to work, but there you have it.

The irony of the situation wasn't lost on me. Here I was, the picture of health in all other ways, stepping on the scale every morning, expecting my body to betray me. When it came to my weight, I'd always treated my body like a criminal that needed constant surveillance. I knew that extreme dieting was madness, but before Jessica's program, I wasn't aware of any other option.

When I first received Jessica's book, I was skeptical that this program, or tapping, would do anything for me or my body. Reading through it, however, I was immediately struck by the research showing that tapping decreases cortisol levels! That's right—the very stress hormone that leads to weight gain is decreased simply by tapping. This was a revelation.

So I decided to try her program in spite of my skepticism—and I was amazed by how quickly it transformed me and my body. Working with Jessica, I realized that I'd been holding on to two limiting beliefs. First, I'd unconsciously bought into the idea that losing weight, exercising, eating right, and feeling good in my body were a struggle for me—and they always would be. Second, I'd gotten caught up in our cultural belief that our worth as women is closely tied to our weight. I could never be slim enough; there was always another five or ten pounds to lose. When it came to weight loss, enough was never enough, which prevented me from ever feeling confident in my own body.

With Jessica's guidance, using tapping to clear the anxiety that was distorting my relationship with my body, my beliefs began to transform. The first and most noticeable change was how I felt about exercise. Since childhood, I'd seen exercise as a chore. Nearly every family outing I can remember—starting at the age of 4—involved carrying heavy gear up a mountain. Seriously, I climbed Mt. Washington in ski boots at the age of 10 while hauling my skis, poles, and a backpack. It was grueling! Those early experiences had left me with the belief that exercise was something I could never enjoy, so I was shocked (and delighted!) when, as a result of this program, I just woke up every morning and wanted to exercise. I now look forward to moving my body. Exercise has become a true source of pleasure for me. Not a necessary chore. What a shift!

Using tapping regularly, I also decided to skip the crash diet and enjoy taking care of myself instead. Rather than restricting food and weighing myself, I ate fresh foods that I love and began to focus on appreciating the body that I have.

So did I fit into my desired clothing size for my photo shoot? Yes! I could easily zip up each dress and pair of pants I'd planned to wear. For the first time in many years, throughout the day of the photo shoot, I felt incredible. Being so at ease in my body and my clothes has been such a new experience for me, and I've gotten compliment after compliment about how great I look. What a wonderful surprise this has all been!

I have built my career on the belief that our bodies know what they need and that they will tell us what that is. What I now realize is that those messages can come in blurry. They can be obscured by false beliefs about our worthiness, our shortcomings, and our inadequacies. Regular diets are based on these limiting beliefs. They are based on us shutting our bodies up and telling ourselves that we're bad. Regular diets are about forcing our bodies into submission, but let's face it— that doesn't work. Even when you eat very little and exercise a lot, diets don't necessarily work. I've tried them. You've likely tried them. Many will create some quick results, but they're always unsustainable, and they just take you further away from what your body is trying to tell you.

But here's the good news—no matter what you believe, it's possible to transform those beliefs, and as a result, transform your biology. Whether you are addicted to sugar, hate exercise, or think that it's not possible for you to have confidence in your body, your solution is in this book. Through the many tapping sequences you'll find here, plus the online support that Jessica provides, you will find your way back to the body confidence and wisdom that are your personal birthright. It's time we stop the madness of extreme dieting and exercise and create a new relationship with ourselves, our emotions, our food and our bodies—and through that process, transform our bodies in ways that feel natural and pleasurable.

*The Tapping Solution for Weight Loss and Body Confidence* works. Pure and simple. Try a little tapping. You have nothing to lose. Except maybe a few pounds, some outmoded beliefs—and a boatload of excess cortisol.

—CHRISTIANE NORTHRUP, M.D.

# Introduction

For many years, I was sure that losing weight was the answer to all my problems. Once I could fit into that dress or those jeans, I'd be happy, my career would take off, and I'd start dating. But only *after* I'd lost the weight. Only when I no longer looked like . . . *this*.

Until then, I'd continue to panic every time someone took my picture, strategically placing my hands over the parts I hated. Or cropping the picture so only my face showed if my hands weren't big enough to cover those parts.

Until then, I'd cancel plans. I'd shrink emotionally so people wouldn't notice how big I felt physically. I'd continue to buy books on weight loss, exercise equipment, and diet food. One day I'd be happy, but not today, not until I lost this weight.

Does this sound familiar?

Losing weight has become a cultural obsession, made apparent by the fact that weight loss has grown into a billion-dollar industry. My guess is that if you picked up this book, it probably isn't the first time you've paid for something to help you lose weight.

Why does nothing seem to work? Why, when you have such a strong desire to lose weight, do your many attempts to shed the weight for good fall short? There's clearly something missing, some hidden key to having a body you can feel proud of—but what is it? Is it exercising more, or doing a certain kind of exercise? Should you eat all carbs, or none at all? Vegan? High protein? In a world that's constantly overwhelming you with contradictory information, what will finally make the difference in your quest to lose weight?

It can be summed up in two words: your emotions.

Your emotions control your beliefs about yourself, your weight, and your worth. They also control your actions. Have you ever made a plan to eat healthy only to find yourself halfway through a box of cookies, thinking, *Did I really do this . . . again?* Your emotions are the driving force behind every action you take. You may know exactly what you "should" be doing, but you're not doing it because your emotions sidetrack you.

Emotions such as anger, fear, resentment, and guilt that are hijacking your best intentions are also impacting you on a deep biological level. Talking about this is an essential conversation that we're not having. We hear so much about food and exercise, but what about the overproduction of cortisol, known as the "stress hormone," that is directly linked to abdominal obesity? The research is out there, but we've been conditioned to believe that weight loss is only about eating the right foods and exercising more. If we don't succeed, we blame our genes—or worse, we believe that there's something inherently broken about us.

During many years of yo-yo dieting and unsuccessful attempts to keep the weight off, I, too, felt broken. I masked it with my smile and my desire to please everyone around me, but behind closed doors I was crumpling up clean paper towels and placing them in the garbage to cover the wrappers of the multiple candy bars I'd just eaten.

Like so many women who feel ashamed of their bodies and their weight, I was a closet emotional eater. It started when I was young. I remember my first solo binge so clearly. I was only seven, and I was faced with an entire plate covered rim to rim with chocolate chip cookies. I sat on the downstairs couch and ate the entire thing while listening closely to make sure no one was walking down the stairs. Even when I was that young, I already had the belief that what I was doing was shameful.

That plate of cookies was the beginning of a years-long love/hate affair with chocolate and other sugary, and occasionally salty, treats.

For me the cravings were very real physical sensations that quickly overwhelmed my ability to reason with myself, or remember how sick I had felt last time. They came on suddenly and felt like a physical need that I *had to* fulfill. As that habit followed me into puberty, I found myself gaining weight, and then panicking and making desperate attempts to lose it.

For brief periods of time, I devoted my every waking hour to dieting and extreme exercise. Starving myself and working out were my punishments for being fat. After losing a few pounds, I began to relax. Then, as if suffering from amnesia, I turned back to food. *I've been so good. I deserve this!* I told myself. *I'm so stressed out, let me just eat this one thing*, I said to myself. Before long, I found myself looking at my reflection in the mirror, feeling defeated and heartbroken, overwhelmed by hatred, disappointment, and anger.

As Einstein so famously said, insanity is doing the same thing over and over again and expecting a different result. Simply put, I was insane. My diets were insane. Belittling myself, shaming myself, and using guilt in an attempt to help me "get my act together" were all insane.

Fortunately, in 2004 my oldest brother, Nick Ortner, introduced me to tapping, also called EFT tapping, a stress relief technique that involves tapping on acupressure points. Tapping would eventually bring an end to the insanity that had ruled my weight loss and body confidence journey up to that point. To be quite frank, though, when I was first introduced to it, it was tapping itself that seemed insane to me.

The first time Nick showed me what tapping was, I was so sure he was playing a practical joke on me that I refused to play along. When I finally gave in and tried it, I was shocked by how quickly I got results. After just ten minutes of tapping, a sinus cold I had at the time, which had been so severe that it had kept me in bed for two full days, disappeared. I remember being shocked that after tapping I could breathe through my nose again. It seemed like a mini miracle; after I tapped through my physical symptoms—and then through my stress and frustration that my career seemed to be going nowhere—my sinus cold symptoms vanished. It was the first time I realized how severely I had been underestimating the impact of emotions and stress on the body.

A couple of years later, Nick and I, along with his close friend, Nick Polizzi, began making our documentary film, *The Tapping Solution*, which shows real people's results with tapping. The making of the documentary was not only a big risk financially, it also continuously tested the strength of our dream. With zero film experience or outside funding, the only way we could move forward was to deal with our own anxiety and limiting beliefs around what was possible. It may sound cliché, but we were only able to create a film about tapping because we used tapping personally every step of the way.

What is tapping exactly? Stay with me. I'll go into more detail in Chapters 1 and 2.

Although I was making strides in other areas of my life with tapping, during those early years, I never, ever used tapping on the one challenge that had controlled my entire life and happiness since childhood—my weight and body image.

My struggle with weight was a huge part of who I thought I was, but it was also something I felt ashamed of and was always trying to hide. Even when I'd lost the weight after weeks of extreme dieting and exercise, I'd obsess all day long about my weight and what I had or hadn't eaten. Even during my "skinny" phases, I had no peace, no happiness.

My obsession with my weight, I later realized, had blinded me from seeing what was going on beneath the surface. Like so many of the women I now teach and coach, I had been conditioned to believe that losing weight was about willpower. For years I was convinced that I had entered this world without the willpower I was sure skinny people must have. Even after years of studying personal development, rarely, if ever, did I think about how my emotions might be impacting my struggle with weight.

Then, in 2008, something happened that forced me to stop the madness and take a serious look at the pain beneath my weight.

While attending a conference one day, I was approached by a woman who recognized me and immediately began raving about my work. By this point, the movie had come out and thousands of people had heard my interviews online. It was one of the first times I'd met a fan in person, so I was thrilled to hear such positive feedback. After showering me with praise, though, she made a comment that hit me like a bomb. "You're bigger than I thought," she said as she looked me up and down. And just like that, I went from feeling elated and excited to hopeless and deflated.

It was one of many, many times over the years that people had commented on my weight, and finally I had to admit that I needed a new approach. Her judgment hurt me so deeply because I was constantly judging myself. It was time to take a deeper look at my relationship with my body and my weight, not to please others but to finally address the pain I'd been hiding behind my weight. When I returned home after that conference, I began piecing together what I'd learned from the hundreds of tapping experts, personal development gurus, and psychiatrists and psychologists I'd interviewed, and I began applying it to myself.

Before I started using tapping to create a new weight loss experience for myself, I made just a couple of rules: I wasn't allowed to diet or punish myself with extreme exercise. Neither had worked for me in the past, and I couldn't let myself go down that road again. Also, I could no longer use my weight as an excuse not to be happy or go for what I wanted in life. That hadn't worked, either.

I began to look at my relationship with my body, food, and exercise as well as sexual intimacy, pleasure, and perfection, and I realized that I wasn't broken. I just had layers of beliefs that made life *feel* unbearable if I couldn't turn to food for comfort.

It suddenly hit me—it was nearly impossible to take good care of something I hated. I'd spent so long hating my body that I didn't know how to respect and nurture myself or my body. By focusing so much on my exterior, I also robbed myself of the opportunity to feel good about myself and my body, simply because I didn't meet a cultural standard of beauty that is obsessed with thinness. That created stress that interfered with my weight loss and with my own happiness.

Tapping took the edge off so I could continue the process and address the feelings and beliefs that had held me captive for so long.

It also relieved my stress and cleared the emotional baggage that had kept my body stuck in a state of anxiety and stress.

As all of that stress and emotional baggage faded away thanks to tapping, I could finally sense what my body needed to thrive. It was incredibly liberating to choose foods that supported my health and well-being—and take real pleasure in eating them. I also began to look forward to moving my body for the first time in my life.

The more I appreciated and loved my body the way it was, the easier it was to take care of it. I also allowed myself to appreciate my accomplishments, experience pleasure, and feel beautiful, even before I'd lost the weight. Using tapping, I was finally able to begin living my life and stepping into my power. The more I did that, the easier and more effortless weight loss became.

After spending more than ten years putting my happiness on hold because of my weight, I could finally see that I'd had the process backward. Losing weight doesn't give you more confidence; self-confidence leads to weight loss and a stronger, healthier body. For me and the thousands of clients and students I've worked with in recent years, losing weight and gaining body confidence was never about the fat. It was always about how we chose to see ourselves and stand up in the world.

There is great power in awareness, in that moment when we get honest with ourselves and can suddenly see things more clearly. But awareness alone is often not enough. We may know consciously what is holding us back but still experience a disconnect between our thoughts and actions. That is where tapping comes in. I continue to be amazed by the results it produces, not just in me but in the hundreds of thousands of lives we have been honored to touch through our movie, *The Tapping Solution*, our online programs, and the annual Tapping World Summit.

I wasted a lot of time complaining that I had "tried everything" and "nothing works for me." The one thing I hadn't tried was loving and approving of myself. Tapping made that possible, and what followed were incredible results in my body and life.

# About This Book

When I was first asked to write this book, I sat on my kitchen floor and sobbed. I felt panicked by the idea of sharing my journey in such a public way. I also didn't want to be seen as part of the weight loss industry, which, in too many cases, has profited from making women feel bad about themselves. That's not who I am, and that's not the career I want.

The reason I eventually agreed to write it was that I knew that what I wanted to share wasn't what you find in a standard weight loss book. I don't believe in dieting, and I have no exercise plan for you to follow. Instead, I wanted to take women through the same journey of self-discovery and exploration that I took, and that I have guided thousands of clients and students on as well.

While the term "weight loss" is in the title of this book and my online course, the truth is that—provided weight isn't interfering with your health—I'm not that concerned with weight for its own sake. For me, weight loss is a happy side effect of loving yourself more and feeling more powerful and beautiful in your own body. That is what I truly hope women experience from embarking on this journey, because when you feel those things, your entire life opens up. Suddenly, your internal and external realities shift in amazing and inspiring ways, and your dreams begin turning into your reality.

What's funny is that while weight loss is never my top priority, the pounds come off anyway, and very consistently, over and over again in my students and clients. That's really the magic of this process. By using this incredibly powerful tool—tapping—to clear stress and limiting emotions and beliefs, you can very quickly get in touch with what you and your body actually need. You can then put *more* focus on your emotions and your relationship with your body, and *less* focus on actual weight loss. As ironic as it may sound, that is when my clients and students are able to lose the weight and keep it off in a way that feels natural, even effortless.

While the weight loss is amazing, what excites me most is seeing the shift in how women feel and how they begin to live their lives.

Before even losing the weight, women stop hiding; they fall in love with themselves and make great strides in their relationships and their careers; they celebrate their beauty, not just because of a number they see on the scale or in their closets, but because they *feel* beautiful.

As you may have already guessed, the process I share in this book is tailored specifically to women. While tapping is effective for weight loss in both genders, women have a unique experience with weight and body confidence.

I created the methods in this book for my students, and I've learned a lot through teaching them and interacting with them as they work their way through the process. I've tried to address some of their most common questions and issues throughout the book. Here's a quick look at what you'll learn as you work your way through the pages.

In Part I of the book, I'll teach you the basics of tapping, showing you what it is and why it works. Then I'll help launch you on your weight loss and body confidence journey by teaching you how to use this technique to move past the first obstacle many people face—panic. In Part II, I'll walk you through the process of "peeling the onion," looking at the deeper aspects of your weight and body confidence challenges. This will really help you release and clear old patterns and emotions that have interfered with weight loss in the past. And then in Part III, you'll create a more empowering relationship with exercise as well as food, and learn how to implement self-care in your life.

As you read this book and experience this process, I encourage you to do all of the exercises and use all of the tapping meditations. My tapping meditations, which you'll find at the end of most chapters, are designed to help you incorporate what you learned in the chapter. It is crucial that you do the tapping. Without tapping, this process may show you why you've struggled with weight, but it won't consistently deliver the long-term weight loss and body confidence that it does with tapping.

I recommend that you read the book in its entirety once, and then return to the parts that resonate with you. My hope is that you'll come back to this book whenever you need some support. Let it be your companion throughout your journey.

I feel so incredibly honored to be sharing this process with you, and I hope that this is the beginning of your journey toward having a healthy body that you sincerely love and appreciate each and every day. More important, I hope that this is the start of your journey toward truly loving and accepting yourself as the incredible and amazing woman you are. From this point forward, may you see your true worth and value in this world.

# Part I

# Preparing for the Journey

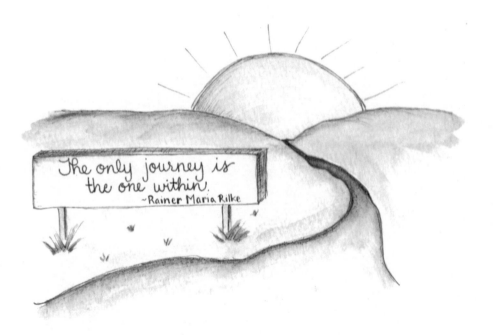

The only journey is
the one within.
~Rainer Maria Rilke

# Chapter 1

# How Tapping Helps You Lose Weight

Standing tall at six feet five, Dawson Church, Ph.D., is a hard man to miss.

I had just walked into a conference in London where Dr. Church and I were both scheduled to speak on tapping. Happy to see him at the other end of the hall, I stood on my tippy toes to wave hello. (At five feet two, I'm rarely in his direct line of sight.)

I'd had the pleasure of working with Dr. Church several times since we first met in 2007 while I was filming *The Tapping Solution*. I'd always appreciated his jovial nature—he has a laugh so jolly, it could make Santa Claus jealous—so I was excited when he excused himself from the crowd that had gathered around him and came rushing over.

Right away I could tell he had something exciting to tell me. After some quick "how's the family?" chitchat, Dr. Church explained that he'd just returned from a medical conference where he'd presented the test results of his latest study for the first time.

He explained that the research had confirmed the science behind what I'd experienced myself and seen in thousands of others—that tapping is an incredibly effective way to decrease the negative impacts of stress on the body.

Dr. Church's research, which I'll share in this chapter, and several other groundbreaking studies help explain why tapping helps us lose weight and keep it off without dieting, deprivation, or extreme exercise.

## Tapping and Weight Loss

Dr. Peta Stapleton is a clinical psychologist in Queensland, Australia, who has spent the past 20 years treating eating disorders in her patients and researching weight loss and specific eating behaviors. At the time of our interview, she had concluded the first (and most important) phase of her study on how tapping impacts food cravings and weight loss. The results were, and still are, incredibly exciting—proof of what I've seen repeatedly in my clients and students.

In doing this study, Dr. Stapleton wanted to find out whether tapping affects weight loss and food cravings, and if so, how effective it is. Because of the weight loss success she and her team had documented in study participants, Dr. Stapleton had actually released some of her findings to the international medical community before they were scheduled to be published.

All of the 89 women in her controlled study were between 31 and 56 years old, and had a body mass index (BMI) that qualified them as being obese. Over an eight-week period, they completed approximately two hours of tapping per week, which averages out to just over 15 minutes per day. Just by doing the tapping—without dieting or exercise—participants lost an average of 16 pounds by the end of the study!

While Dr. Stapleton expected that participants would lose weight from doing the tapping, she admits to being surprised by how much weight these women lost. What's even more exciting is that the weight loss they achieved during the initial eight weeks seemed to last for six or more months afterward, even though most of the study participants stopped tapping once the initial eight-week period ended.

How is that possible? How can tapping lead to such dramatic and lasting weight loss in such a short period of time? To understand Dr. Stapleton's research results, let's first take a look at how stress affects the body.

# Your Body's Weight Gain Cocktail

You have a pharmacy inside you. At all times, your body is pumping out the hormones and chemicals it needs to function properly. Unfortunately, many of us are taking a drug that, in excessive amounts, causes weight gain. We take it daily, and that drug is called stress.

Stress begins in the amygdala, an almond-shaped component located in the limbic system, or midbrain. The amygdala has been called the body's smoke detector. When it senses danger, it tells our brain to initiate a physiological stress response called the fight-or-flight response. This creates an overproduction of a hormone called cortisol, which studies have linked to increased appetite, sugar cravings, and added abdominal fat. Even mild stress, like worrying about why your jeans feel too tight or that you'll never lose the baby weight, can cause your body to go into the fight-or-flight response. This same stress response happens when you experience common negative emotions like anger, fear, and guilt.

The fight-or-flight response prepares the body for danger, getting it ready to either fight off an attacker or take flight, as our ancient ancestors had to do when they encountered a tiger in the wild. Since this stress response was intended to save you from an immediate threat, all of your body's defense systems are quickly activated. Your adrenaline levels increase, your muscles tighten, and your blood pressure, heart rate, and blood sugar all rise so that you can react quicker, run faster, and climb higher.

Because all of your body's energy is being channeled toward self-defense, less essential functions such as digestion are either slowed down or shut down altogether. (Indigestion doesn't register as an urgent issue when you're literally running for your life!) But that inability to digest food properly and efficiently has a negative impact on your metabolism and prevents your body from absorbing the nutrients it desperately needs. Without essential nutrients and nourishment, your body may then trigger a feeling of hunger, not because it actually needs more food, but because the stress response has rendered it unable to properly digest the food that *is* available.

Unlike our ancestors, we are subject to a complex assortment of stimuli and stressors that means our stress levels remain higher for longer periods of time, and this means that our bodies are in the fight-or-flight response more frequently and for longer periods of time. That creates more potential for negative effects on our digestion, metabolism, and hormones on an ongoing basis.

So even if you're exercising and eating right, stress can disrupt your weight loss efforts. This is where tapping becomes such a powerful tool. What tapping does incredibly well is disrupt the fight-or-flight response, quickly allowing your body to return to a more relaxed state in which it can digest food properly and support healthier digestion and faster metabolism. Let's take a look at how this happens.

## How Tapping Lowers Your Stress

In a randomized controlled study—the gold standard of scientific research—conducted by Dr. Church (the jovial giant you may recall from earlier), he and his team focused on the changes in cortisol levels and psychological symptoms in 83 subjects. The study participants were divided into three groups: one group was led through an hour-long tapping session, another group received an hour of conventional talk therapy, and a third control group received no treatment.

While the control group and talk therapy group showed only a 14 percent drop of cortisol over time, the tapping group showed a 24 percent decrease in cortisol levels, on average, with some experiencing as much as a 50 percent decrease in cortisol.

The dramatic drop in cortisol in the tapping group was so significant that the lab initially believed there was either something wrong with the samples or with its equipment. To ensure accuracy, it delayed the results by several weeks in order to recalibrate its equipment and run the tests again. After running them repeatedly and getting consistent results, it finally released them to Dr. Church.

In addition to having been rigorously checked and rechecked by the lab, Dr. Church's research findings support earlier research conducted at Harvard Medical School over the last decade. The Harvard studies show that stimulating selected meridian acupoints decreases activity in the amygdala, as well as other parts of the brain associated with negative emotions. In fMRI and PET brain scans, you can clearly see the amygdala's alarm bells being quieted when acupoints are stimulated.

Although the Harvard research focused on stimulating meridian acupoints with needles (acupuncture), a separate double-blind study confirmed the same positive impact when acupoints were stimulated without needles—which is what happens during tapping.

Tapping on acupoints while sorting through emotional challenges is part of an emerging field known as "energy psychology." Much of the existing research in energy psychology is getting more and more attention, partly because it compares favorably to standards set by the Society of Clinical Psychology (Division 12 of the American Psychological Association) as an "evidence-based" approach.

While many psychologists and other mental health professionals are beginning to incorporate tapping into their practice, what my brother and I are so passionate about is the ability everyone has at their own fingertips to experience relief. Once you know tapping, you always have a tool to support you through times of stress. It's incredibly self-empowering.

If you're interested in reading more about dozens of other studies that have demonstrated how effective tapping is for a wide range of disorders and conditions, you can visit www.TheTappingSolution.com/science-and-research.php or check out my brother Nick's *New York Times* best-selling book *The Tapping Solution: A Revolutionary System for Stress-Free Living*.

## A Groundbreaking Discovery

Now that we've looked at some of the more recent science indicating how tapping impacts weight loss and stress, I'd like to share a brief history of tapping, which also shows how effective tapping is at improving overall health and wellness.

It was 1979 when Dr. Roger Callahan, a traditionally trained psychologist, experienced his first major breakthrough using tapping with a patient. It came after he studied the body's meridian points, which are the basis of the ancient Chinese medical technique known as acupuncture. The meridians in the body are energy channels that carry our vital life force, our *qi*, to the various organs and systems in the body. They run up and down both sides of the body, and each meridian is linked to a separate organ—stomach, gallbladder, kidney, and so on. You can access the energy in each meridian through its "endpoint," a specific location on the body's surface.

These "meridian endpoints" are where acupuncture needles are inserted and also where we tap to balance or increase the energy flow within a specific meridian. They're also places we often touch unconsciously during moments of stress—for example, our forehead, chin, and collarbone—perhaps as a way to calm ourselves down.

When he experienced success in using tapping with patients, Dr. Callahan continued his study of meridian points, focusing on merging traditional psychotherapy with tapping. Over time he developed a set of "algorithms," or tapping sequences, to address different issues. For instance, he created one tapping sequence to treat fear and a separate sequence to treat anger. He eventually began teaching his tapping sequences to students.

One of his students, a man named Gary Craig, began experimenting with tapping and discovered that it was the tapping itself rather than the specific sequences that was so effective. To simplify the process, Gary created a single tapping sequence, which has since become the basis of what he later called EFT, or Emotional Freedom Techniques. Many different approaches to tapping are based on Gary Craig's EFT model. Tapping and meridian tapping are the generic names used.

The EFT sequence Gary pioneered includes all of the major meridian endpoints and can be used for all issues. The EFT sequence, which we'll explore in detail in Chapter 2, begins with the side of the hand, then moves to the inner eyebrow, the outer eyebrow, underneath the eye, under the nose, the chin, the collarbone, the side of the rib cage, and finally, the top of the head.

During the same period of time when Craig was simplifying his tapping sequence, Dr. Patricia Carrington, a psychologist and then faculty member at the Department of Psychology at Princeton University, was independently using a single algorithm method and seeing great results in her clients. She created the Choices Method, which we'll explore shortly.

As Gary Craig's and Dr. Carrington's work began to spread, their results caught the attention of psychologists and researchers who have since given us a far better understanding of how tapping helps retrain your brain.

## Retraining Your Brain

To understand why tapping works so well—not just for anxiety, fear, and trauma but also for losing weight—it's important to understand the *limbic response*.

The limbic system is the part of our brain that contains that feisty amygdala that initiates the fight-or-flight response when it senses danger. This same process can take place when we experience stress around food. For instance, when you experience a craving for chocolate, you may be in the throes of a limbic response. If your brain has been trained to respond to stress by inhaling a box of chocolate chip cookies, that's probably what you'll do after a long day at the office.

Because tapping quickly halts the fight-or-flight response and lowers your cortisol levels, you're able to change how your brain reacts to stress and chocolate chip cookies. Instead of being made to feel like you must devour every last one of those cookies, you can stop and figure out whether cookies are really the best way to unwind.

If you have intense food cravings, the idea of being able to pause and determine whether you really want or need to eat the food you're craving may sound impossible. As someone who used to inhale a box of six organic cereal bars in one sitting (a favorite during one of my "healthy eating" phases), I completely understand why you feel that way. In those moments when you feel like you'll die if you don't eat that food, you're at the mercy of a limbic response that's been ingrained in your brain, probably for many years.

The idea that you can train your limbic system to respond differently to familiar stimuli lines up with recent discoveries about *neuroplasticity*, which shows that the brain's pathways can be altered. Scientists speculate that when we train our limbic system to respond to a long day at work in a new way, we're actually changing our neural pathways, training our brain to react differently than it has in the past.

After working with thousands of clients on food cravings and emotional eating, I'm still amazed at how quickly tapping can change behavior. After tapping on the stress they're feeling, clients will often say, "Wow, it's actually not about the food." Once we use tapping to clear the stress that's causing them to overeat, they're able to eat less without even noticing. The situations or foods that once triggered them to overeat simply lose their power.

Does that mean they'll never succumb to cravings and emotional eating ever again? No. But it happens so infrequently that it doesn't sabotage their goals. They often describe finally feeling a sense of peace around food. For the first time in years, clients tell me they can attend parties and have great conversations with people they'd never gotten to know previously because all they could focus on was the food. And for the first time in years, they can take a walk or go to a yoga class and actually enjoy themselves.

The success stories around tapping, weight loss, and body confidence cover a wide range of circumstances, issues, and challenges. Whatever the specifics of the story, time after time when clients do the tapping, they lose the weight and keep it off. More important, though, even before the weight loss happens, they're able to feel beautiful in their bodies.

# Why Tap When You Just Want to Lose Weight Now?

People often ask me how quickly tapping will help them lose weight. While many of my clients begin losing weight in our first weeks working together, everyone loses weight at their own pace. When we begin tapping to release the stress and pressure we put on ourselves to lose weight, it's counterproductive to obsess about the result. When we are truly on this journey, weight loss becomes a pleasurable side effect of feeling better about ourselves.

The great thing about tapping is that it also works on headaches, backaches, and almost any kind of physical pain as well as insomnia and negative emotions such as fear, anger, and more. You can use it to relax after a long day or to get more focused when you're feeling sluggish. The physical and emotional benefits are endless, so try tapping whenever you want to feel better, and the weight loss benefits will soon appear as well.

# Anyone Can Lose Weight with Tapping

As compelling as the science around tapping is, for me it's the incredible results I've seen in my clients, myself, and my friends and family that offer the real proof that tapping is the most powerful weight loss tool I've ever seen.

When I began this process, I was a huge skeptic, and to this day I'm amazed at how well tapping works for weight loss, weight maintenance, body confidence, stress, illness, physical pain, and so much more. But over the years, I've become passionate about tapping as a health and weight loss tool because the results I see are so undeniable. My skepticism had no choice but to admit defeat.

Many clients I work with start out with this same skepticism. I always appreciate that they're honest with me about it. Just like me, they'd already tried countless other methods to lose weight—diets, extreme exercise, hypnosis, meditation. And with each new attempt at losing weight, they'd either see no change or lose it only to gain it right back. Why would tapping be any different?

But once they start, they lose the weight, not because they're dieting but because they learn to live life and be happy in the moment. Tapping helps decrease your cortisol levels, so your hormones can support your weight loss. Tapping also supports you in sticking with healthy lifestyle changes. I'll share many client stories throughout this book, and the people in them are living proof that you don't have to believe that tapping will help you lose weight for the tapping to work. Whether or not you believe it will work for you, if you do the tapping, you can achieve all of your weight loss goals and keep the weight off. So let's get started tapping.

# Chapter 2

# Quick Start Tapping Guide

Nancy's stress levels were at an all-time high. A 53-year-old entrepreneur trying to run her business while relocating from New York City to San Francisco, she stepped on the scale one day while packing the contents of her bathroom. She was horrified to see that she was at her highest weight ever. This wasn't the first time she'd felt surprised and heartbroken while looking at the scale.

Nancy had trouble remembering a time when she wasn't stressed about her weight. She ran the pattern of starting the latest diet trend, working hard, losing some weight, and then gaining it back. When she did manage to lose weight, she often felt like "the wolves were at my door," as she put it. One false move around food and she'd be back to her old ways of eating, and then she'd regain the weight.

As she began her new adventure in San Francisco, she decided she was ready to leave her pattern of chronic dieting and stress in New York. "I kept saying to myself that there had to be another way. I wanted to end this pattern." Nancy had heard me speak at an event and soon learned that her brother had been using tapping to manage stress. When she heard about my weight loss program, she decided to take a leap of faith and signed up for it in the midst of her move.

By the time Nancy was settled in San Francisco, she had been tapping for four months, often using my tapping meditations. Although moving was stressful, she was able to use tapping to find relief every step of the way. When she finally got around to unpacking her scale, she was surprised once again—pleasantly surprised! She had lost weight during a time when she was unable (and unwilling) to follow a strict diet plan.

I came across Nancy's story because she was so thrilled by her results that she decided to blog about it on a website for female entrepreneurs. This is what she wrote:

> I no longer crave sugar, sweets, and carbs. I rarely eat them and don't miss them one bit. And when I do, I savor a small portion guilt free, and it's not a big deal. All the drama around food, weight, and body image has simply been unplugged. I've also lost 16 pounds, pretty effortlessly, I might add! And, most important, now I really understand how stressing about dieting and weight—and especially negative self-talk—only fuels the problem. Finally I get what I've been doing wrong all these years! This is the only program I've ever found that nails the emotional stuff that is really at the root of it all.

Are you ready to "nail" the emotional stuff like Nancy did? It begins with learning how to tap.

## Let's Start Tapping!

First let me just say that if you're new to tapping, I understand that it seems weird. Here's how I think of it. You know those times when you try to think yourself out of a thought? You're an intelligent, self-aware person, and you feel like you should be able to use positive reasoning to get rid of that thought or emotion, but you can't because you feel it in your body. It might be anxiety in your chest or a panicked feeling in your stomach. What tapping does is bridge that gap between your body and your mind. When you tap while focusing on the thought or feeling, you relax the body and send a calming signal to the brain, telling it that it, too, can relax.

In addition to its effectiveness, one of the reasons my clients have such success with tapping is that it works so well with their busy schedules. It's easy, convenient, and makes you feel great in a matter of minutes. So let's dive right in. Here are the basic steps for tapping:

- Step 1: Choose your tapping target, and create a reminder phrase (see pages 15–19).

- Step 2: Rate the intensity of your target on the 0 to 10 Subjective Units of Distress Scale (SUDS; see pages 19–20).

- Step 3: Create a setup statement (see page 21).

- Step 4: Tap on the karate chop point (see page 22) while repeating your setup statement three times.

- Step 5: Tap gently through the eight points in the tapping sequence (see pages 22–24) while saying your reminder phrase out loud. Tap five to seven times on each point. Repeat this until you begin to feel relief.

- Step 6: Once you're feeling better, take a deep breath and again rate the intensity of your issue using the 0 to 10 SUDS.

It's that simple! I'll lead you through the process in more detail in the rest of this chapter; however, if you're a visual learner, you can watch a video on how to tap where I cover all of the steps. You can find that video at www.TheTappingSolution.com/chapter2.

## Step 1: Pinpointing Your Tapping Target

You're reading this book, so it seems safe to assume that you're anxious to lose weight and feel more confident in your body. Like many women, though, you're probably living a full life, perhaps juggling work, family, and friends, maybe also trying to manage physical pain or illness, and stressed about your finances or the fight you just had with your boss or husband. Whatever issue is bothering you most is a great place to start with your tapping target.

It might be one of these:

- *Work has been really stressful lately.*

- *I'm so frustrated about my weight.*

- *I have a really bad headache.*

Take a moment to answer these questions for yourself: *What's really bothering me right now? What in my life feels really stressful right now?* You can either write it down or just remember it as you continue reading. Keep in mind, too, that your list doesn't have to seem relevant to weight loss and body confidence. Very often the stress that impacts our weight doesn't appear at first to be directly related to weight.

If several different issues come to mind, just start with the one that feels the most stressful. There's no right or wrong answer, so just go with whichever issue comes to mind first or feels most pressing right now.

Once you've got your tapping target and have started tapping, you'll want to get as specific as possible. For example, if work is your top source of stress right now, why is it so stressful? Do you feel like your boss never appreciates your work? Have you recently started a new job or business?

Tapping on a general issue can certainly improve your mood and make you feel better. But adding specific details—like the fact that you just saw a recent photo of yourself and you feel ashamed of how big you think you look in it—draws the focus more clearly to what you're experiencing. By being as specific as possible, you'll be better able to rewire the brain's response to whatever is causing your stress. You'll notice that you can still have the thought but without feeling physical anxiety in your body. This is when you'll be able to relax and choose a better thought or action.

If you ever get stuck on what to say, just focus on the feeling. You can also visualize a picture of what happened (or is happening) and then describe it as you're tapping. Do whatever it takes to get a clear memory or feeling while you're tapping.

- Here's an example of a broad tapping statement around being stressed about weight: *I'm so stressed about my weight.*

- A more specific tapping statement would be: *I'm so stressed about my weight because I just saw a recent picture of myself.*

- And an even more specific statement would be: *I'm so stressed about my weight because I saw a recent picture of myself and felt angry at myself for how big I look.*

You can get specific in many different ways. Sometimes focusing on the intensity of the emotion you're experiencing is helpful. For example:

*I'm angry at myself for how big I look in that picture.*
*How angry do I feel? So angry!*
*What would that be on a 0 to 10 scale? Ten!*
*Where do I feel the anger in my body? My stomach—it makes me feel sick just thinking about it.*

Now you have specific details about the anger you're feeling, how angry you feel, where you feel the anger in your body, and so forth. You can use a similar process for physical pain, focusing on exactly where your head hurts, when the headache started, and so on. Whatever the issue, always try to be as specific as possible.

CHOOSING A REMINDER PHRASE

The reminder phrase is short—just a couple of words that bring to mind your tapping target. You will speak this phrase out loud or in your mind at each of the eight points in the tapping sequence. For example, if your tapping target has to do with your feelings of anger

## Finding Your Words

When people first begin tapping, they often tell me they "never know what to say." To help you break through this obstacle, throughout the book I'll give you sample statements you can use for your tapping target. I'll point out common themes I've seen in myself and in my clients, but only you can determine what is really relevant for you at any given moment. You and your life are unique, so whenever you're tapping, I encourage you to tailor your language to your own experiences. There are no right or wrong answers with tapping. The best thing you can do is to trust your instincts. If you do that and follow the process I've laid out, it's nearly impossible to get tapping wrong.

about that picture of yourself, you might tap through each point in the sequence saying, "This anger. . . this anger. . . this anger . . ." Other examples of reminder phrases for different tapping targets might be:

This loneliness I'm feeling . . .
This frustration . . .
This back pain . . .
And so forth.

You're repeating the reminder phrase to remind yourself of the issue at each point. You want to target the thought that's creating the physical discomfort in your body. This reminder phrase serves to keep your focus on the target so you don't get distracted. It also acts as a barometer, helping you determine along the way how true the target feels to you.

Once you get used to tapping, you can change your reminder phrase as you tap through each point. For example, you might say, "This anger . . . this burning anger . . . I feel it in my stomach . . . I feel so humiliated . . ." You will notice that the reminder phrase becomes more specific as you say it. In the meditations at the end of each chapter, I

## My Guided Tapping Meditations

Years ago while working with a client who was suffering from insomnia, I recorded a tapping audio to help her sleep. The recording helped her so much that I created more of them to share with as many people as possible.

I've since recorded many different tapping audios, which I call "tapping meditations." People have found them to be very useful starting points for getting comfortable with tapping, which is great. The goal with tapping, however, is always to be as specific as possible, so while my tapping meditations can be useful tools, I always encourage people to tap in response to their own experiences, being as specific as possible about what they're experiencing at any given moment.

To download a copy of a morning and evening tapping meditation for weight loss, visit www.TheTappingSolution.com/chapter2.

provide a tapping meditation that evolves in this way. Feel free to use these tapping meditations as prompts and then tailor them specifically to your experience and emotions. To begin, though, you can focus on keeping it simple by saying the same statement at each point.

## Step 2: Using SUDS, the 0 to 10 Scale

Now that you're aware of your tapping target, I want you to give it a number on the 0 to 10 SUDS, or Subjective Units of Distress Scale.

Think about your tapping target and notice what it brings up in your body. What level of distress does it generate in you? A 10 would be the most distress you can imagine; a 0 rating would mean you don't feel any distress at all. Don't worry about getting the SUDS level exact or "right"— just follow your gut instinct. Think about the anger you feel as a result of how you look in that picture. If the feeling is really intense, you might

> Self-acceptance is an invitation to stop trying to change yourself into the person you wish to be, long enough to find out who you really are.
>
> —ROBERT HOLDEN

rate it an 8 or a 9. If you're still feeling anger toward yourself but the intensity has lessened a bit since you first saw the photo, you might rate it a 5 or 6. To see a significant shift in an issue, start with something you can rate at 5 or higher.

SUDS is best used to measure emotional intensity, and there are two main reasons we use it. First, when we clear an issue with tapping, we sometimes experience so much relief that we forget how intense the issue was before tapping. Also, by using SUDS we're able to appreciate the progress we're making through tapping. It's not always a necessary step, but it can be very helpful.

## Do I Have to Say "I Love and Accept Myself"?

When I teach tapping to a new crowd, I can see the restlessness in the audience as I begin to talk about the setup statement. For many it feels incredibly uncomfortable and even a bit "out there" to say "I love and accept myself," especially when this is the opposite of how they may be feeling. I can relate. I used to think that people who said it were either narcissistic or just plain corny. But I soon learned the incredible power of this phrase.

We have been taught that in order to achieve something, we need to fight for it. Accepting ourselves supposedly means we surrender to our flaws and never change. But it's our inability to accept ourselves that keeps us stuck in place. We are so busy fighting our feelings that we don't realize that the very act of fighting or trying to ignore negative feelings gives them power over us.

When we don't accept how we feel, we pile on even more emotions. Have you ever been upset at yourself for being upset? *I'm so mad at myself*

## Step 3: Creating Your Setup Statement

Now that you know your SUDS level, the next step is to craft what's called the "setup statement." This brings up the energy of the tapping target you're going to be working on. The basic setup statement goes like this:

Even though _____ [fill in the blank with your tapping target], I love and accept myself.

So you might say, "Even though I feel ashamed at how big I look in that picture, I love and accept myself" or "Even though my head is pounding, I love and accept myself" or "Even though I'm stressed out about this work deadline, I love and accept myself."

*for being mad! I should know better by now and not let him/her trigger me like this!* When we don't accept how we feel, we keep that emotion stuck in place, and over time the pile of emotions we're stuck with gets bigger and bigger. Loving and accepting ourselves releases us from this pattern and gives us the freedom to choose a more empowering thought. Again and again I have seen the profound impact of acceptance. It is the first step to true transformation. As my friend Kris Carr says, "When we truly embrace acceptance, that's when our body exhales and can begin healing."

Still resistant to this concept? While I always encourage people to try saying "I love and accept myself," another statement I often use is "Even though I feel so [fill in the blank], I accept how I feel and I'm okay." You can also use EFT expert Dr. Patricia Carrington's Choices Method of countering the emotion you're feeling and adding "and I choose . . ." at the end. For example, if you're feeling overwhelmed, you could use the setup statement "Even though I'm feeling overwhelmed, I choose to feel calm and confident."

## Step 4: Tap on the Karate Chop Point

To begin the physical process of tapping, start by tapping on the karate chop point (see the illustration on page 23) while you repeat your setup statement three times. The same meridians run down both sides of the body, so you can tap with either hand, on whichever side of the body feels best to you.

## Step 5: Tapping Through the Points

After the karate chop, you are ready to start tapping through the eight points of the tapping sequence, also shown in the illustration on page 23, while repeating your reminder phrase. These points are

- Eyebrow

- Side of Eye

- Under Eye

- Under Nose

- Chin

- Collarbone

- Under Arm

- Top of Head

Just as with the karate chop point, you can tap the point on either side of your body. You can also tap both sides at once if you'd like (it's not necessary, however, because you'll hit the same meridian lines regardless of which side you tap). Aim for tapping five to seven times

# Tapping Points

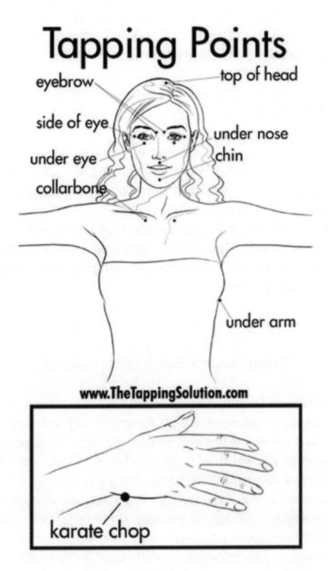

eyebrow

top of head

side of eye

under nose

under eye

chin

collarbone

under arm

www.TheTappingSolution.com

karate chop

at each stop as you work through the sequence, but it doesn't have to be an exact count. If it feels right to tap 20 times—or 100—on one point, do it! The idea is simply to spend enough time at that point to speak your reminder phrase and let it sink in.

## Step 6: Check In

Now that you've completed a round of tapping, take a deep breath. Feel your body and notice what's happening for you. Ask yourself these questions: *Did the issue shift? What thoughts came up for me while tapping? How do I feel on the 0 to 10 scale now?*

Go back and think about the issue and see how it feels to you now. You might find that the intensity of your emotions has decreased. In that case, you can tap a few more rounds using the same language and clear the issue altogether.

### When Should I Switch to the Positive?

The main goal with tapping is to lower the stress you have around certain thoughts. It's important to focus on the negative so you can process how you feel. This is always the first and most crucial step. Then, when you feel that the intensity is lower than 5, you can begin to incorporate how you would like to feel instead. This isn't a necessary step but I find it very helpful. Only use positive affirmations if they feel true when you tap. If you find yourself resisting an empowering thought, continue focusing on how you really feel and keep tapping. Remember, tapping sends that calming signal to the brain letting your brain know it's safe to relax. When you relax while thinking of a negative thought, it's easier to process the feeling, change your mind, and pick another thought. The relaxation response also makes it easier to accept those positive thoughts that feel good and relaxing.

At times you'll find that, for example, as you were tapping on your anger over how you looked in that picture, another memory or feeling came up. This often happens, and it's actually good news. Just keep tapping on issues that come up. Through this process you "peel the onion," revealing layer after layer of an issue so that, over time, you can create a new relationship with yourself and your body.

My advice is to keep tapping until your tapping target finds enough relief that you feel noticeably better. This may mean getting the SUDS level down to a 2 or 3, which may seem manageable to you, or it may mean clearing it altogether so it's at 0. Tap long enough to release your pain, whether it's physical, emotional, or spiritual. Stick with it. Do five rounds; do ten rounds. Whenever possible, commit to getting the relief you need.

Are you ready to give it a try? Start by saying your setup statement three times while tapping on the karate chop point. Then move on to tap your reminder phrase at each of the eight points in the sequence—eyebrow, side of eye, under eye, under nose, chin, collarbone, under arm, and top of head. Don't worry about getting it perfect the first time around; what matters is that you start tapping! Remember to visit www.TheTappingSolution.com/chapter2 if you need additional support to get started.

## Tapping Through the Layers

We began the tapping example by talking about the anger you might feel when looking at a photo. Tapping on an emotion is one way to begin the process of clearing the obstacles that keep you from losing weight. However, as I mentioned earlier, we use a "peel the onion" approach when we tap to address the various layers of any given issue. As we just saw, sometimes you start with one target—anger—and then find something else underneath it.

When an issue has multiple layers, you may need to address each one in order to fully clear the issue. Working through these layers might seem tedious at first, but the reality is that emotional and physical experiences are often multilayered. Remember: you don't need to do it all at once. Be gentle with yourself.

So how do you know which target to choose to start your exploration with tapping? The four most common types of targets to work with are symptoms/side effects, emotions, events, and limiting beliefs. We'll cover each one of these next.

## The Tapping Tree: Identify Your Targets

Originally created by EFT master Lindsay Kenny, the Tapping Tree is a wonderful metaphor to help you understand the interconnection between all the pieces of the weight loss puzzle. The roots of the tree are our limiting beliefs—what we believe to be true or not true about ourselves and the world. The trunk represents past events, often traumatic, that still affect us today. The branches are the emotions that come up, including things like shame, frustration, and hopelessness. Finally, the leaves are the side effects or external symptoms that manifest and add to our stress. Keep in mind that we're not saying that everything starts with a limiting belief. You may have experienced an event that later resulted in a limiting belief about yourself or the world.

Throughout the rest of the book we'll tap on all the points of the Tapping Tree. While we tend to want to focus solely on losing the weight, in order to have the kind of long-term weight loss we want, we need to address the underlying issues that have shaped our relationship with ourselves, our body, our weight, and the food we eat.

So often, clients come to me saying that they just need to lose the weight. As we tap together, they remember events—whether from childhood, a divorce, or some other powerful experience—and realize that the pain of that event led to their weight gain and their subsequent struggle with the scale. Others discover that they've been holding on to a belief—that they'll never be good enough, or that weight loss has to be a struggle—and realize that their belief has been preventing them from losing weight.

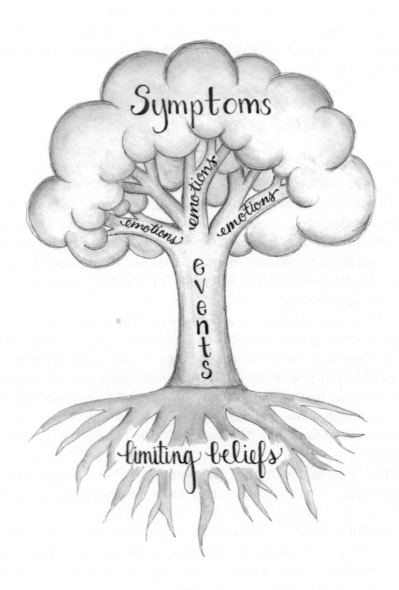

Sometimes you can handle more than one part of the tree at once. For example, by tapping on a "root" limiting belief, you may also clear a "leaf" symptom or side effect. That's what happens when you tap around your stress. Let's go a bit more deeply into each element of the Tapping Tree.

## SYMPTOMS AND SIDE EFFECTS (LEAVES)

Difficulty losing weight and keeping it off, avoiding exercise, cravings, constantly snacking—these are all symptoms or side effects. They can be classified into two areas: physical symptoms and behaviors. Symptoms and side effects are often the most bothersome and the easiest to identify because they are so real and present. While they may seem to be problems in themselves, they are often just expressions of a deeper issue. Ideally, over time you will identify the deeper issue and use that as your tapping target.

That said, tapping on an obvious symptom or side effect is a great starting point—and this can produce excellent results on its own. It can work very well for cravings. For example, if you're craving chocolate, you might use a setup statement like "Even though I really want to eat that box of chocolate, I deeply and completely accept myself." You would tap through the points using reminder words and phrases like "chocolate," "this craving for chocolate," and so forth.

Just by doing this kind of "symptom tapping," many people find that their craving goes away. One student shared her experience with this:

I SERIOUSLY LOVE TWIZZLERS! I have loved them since I was a little girl. My high school boyfriends would "woo" me with pound-sized bags of them. Yesterday afternoon, my son was asleep on the couch. Next to him on the table was a giant sack o' piñata candy from a party last week . . . I found myself peering into the sack, looking for my beloved Twizzlers. None in there. :( But! I remembered there might be a bag way up on the refrigerator. My mouth literally began to salivate. All I could think of was ripping open that bag, smelling that wonderful Twizzler smell, and eating one after another. I made a beeline for the kitchen. But! As I got to the fridge, I diverted to the living room, where I sat on the couch and tapped about HOW BAD I WANTED TO SNARF TWIZZLERS!! Suddenly, I did not want those Twizzlers. I was almost in shock! I actually TRIED to want the Twizzlers, but by that point, I couldn't have cared less about them. Amazing!

When symptom tapping doesn't get the job done, however, that usually means you need to go further down the Tapping Tree to identify a deeper target that will provide the relief you're looking for. A good next step is to look at your emotional state.

## EMOTIONS (BRANCHES)

If you tap on a chocolate craving and the craving persists, you can ask yourself, *What was I feeling when I began craving chocolate?* If, for example, you were angry about something your husband said to you, you can tap on that emotion until it has been cleared. Sometimes you may realize you're feeling several emotions. Different aspects of the target may appear, so what starts as anger might move into hurt and sadness, then into grief and loneliness. If you know that you're experiencing intense emotions, you can begin your tapping with what you're feeling rather than with the symptom or side effect.

Sometimes it's easy to get stuck on the emotions we're most familiar with. For example, many of us end up tapping on feelings of anger and sadness, which are easy to recognize. But accessing a broader range of emotions can help bring more specificity to tapping. Here are some key emotions many of us experience. You can use this list to further connect with what's going on for you.

| | | | |
|---|---|---|---|
| Alienation | Distress | Guilt | Loneliness |
| Ambivalence | Doubt | Hatred | Paranoia |
| Anger | Dread | Homesickness | Pity |
| Anxiety | Embarrassment | Hope | Rage |
| Bitterness | Envy | Hostility | Regret |
| Boredom | Fear | Humiliation | Remorse |
| Contempt | Frustration | Hunger | Resentment |
| Depression | Fury | Hysteria | Shame |
| Despair | Grief | Insecurity | Suffering |
| Disgust | Grouchiness | Loathing | Worry |

## PAST EVENTS (TRUNK)

Another common category of tapping target is past events. There are two kinds: those that happen and are easy to move beyond, and those that affect us and stay with us. The difference between the two kinds of events is whether or not we have processed them emotionally, energetically, and/or physically.

One person can think back to something that happened in grade school—being scolded by a teacher—and be able to say, "Yeah, I remember feeling embarrassed that she singled me out like that, but it doesn't bother me anymore." The memory is there but it doesn't have the emotional charge it once did. The next person thinks about being scolded in grade school and has a totally different experience. She feels it in her gut; when she recalls that moment, intense feelings of embarrassment, anger, and hurt come up. This is an experience that hasn't been processed. Addressing that past event with tapping will help her let go of the pain and move on.

## LIMITING BELIEFS (ROOTS)

Limiting beliefs are misleading conclusions we make about ourselves and the world based on events or experiences. For example, someone might have a limiting belief about her ability to lose weight and keep it off because her weight has fluctuated so much for so many years. As a result, she anticipates that the same pattern will repeat itself in the future, and that belief limits her expectations of what's possible.

It can be hard to see our own limiting beliefs because, to us, they just seem like "the truth." For example, you may believe you'll never lose the baby weight after you have a child because your mom and your sisters never did. As a result of that belief, you may stop exercising because you think, *It's hopeless so what's the point?*

Most of us begin unintentionally collecting limiting beliefs during childhood and then keep adding more as we get older. Parents, teachers, and peers often pass them on to us in our early years and from there they color how we see ourselves, our lives, and others. The belief that "I'll never lose the weight" has profound implications for what and how we eat, whether or not we exercise, even how much effort we make in our relationships and career. That single limiting belief changes how we behave.

Tapping on childhood or past events will often clear limiting beliefs, but when you're aware of a limiting belief, you can also tap directly on that belief.

> Why don't you start believing that no matter what you have or haven't done, that your best days are still out in front of you.
>
> **—JOEL OSTEEN**

## Creating Your Own Tapping Tree

The Tapping Tree is a great visual tool for figuring out what's going on in your life and systematically working through various challenges. It also makes it easier to see how a symptom might be connected to an emotion, event, or belief—how the "leaf" relates to the "branch," "trunk," or "roots." These connections and insights are vital for you to get the best results with tapping. As I'll continue to remind you, it's crucial that you get specific when you tap so you can really focus on what's happening, and the best way to do that is to dig deeper.

As you go through the process laid out in this book, you may want to return to the Tapping Tree and create your own as you discover new

### Is Tapping Too Negative?

Clients sometimes mention their concern that tapping focuses too much on negative thoughts and emotions such as fear, anger, blame, and shame. While I understand their concern, the fact is that we all experience negative emotions. By trying to ignore negative feelings or judge ourselves for having them, we simply give them permission to control us and our behavior unconsciously. If we're angry, for instance, we can't just decide to stop feeling anger by ignoring that feeling. We need to directly address the anger, to somehow "blow off steam," before we can relax and calm down. Tapping gives us an incredibly fast and effective way to address our negative thoughts and emotions so we can once again relax and feel good. The best way to experience less negativity is to tap on the negative aspects of your life—your stress about your weight, your frustration with your boss, your finances, your relationship, and so on. As you tap and clear those negative thoughts and emotions, you'll be able to do tapping using positive statements, which will further lower your stress and improve your ability to lose weight.

tapping targets. You can print out a blank copy of the Tapping Tree drawing by visiting www.TheTappingSolution.com/chapter2. Or you can simply sketch it on a piece of paper. It doesn't have to be pretty; just be sure to leave plenty of space.

## Ready to Lower Your Stress and Start Losing Weight?

Clients often tell me how much they end up enjoying the time they spend tapping each day. Although it feels a bit strange when they're first learning how to tap, they find that they're more relaxed and in a better mood after they spend some time tapping.

The best way to get started with your weight loss journey is to take 15 minutes to begin tapping right now on whatever is causing you stress or anxiety, whether or not it seems related to your weight. Just imagine waking up in the not-so-distant future and feeling great in your body. What would that be like?

Every moment you spend tapping counts, so take the time now to learn the tapping points and practice the process for long enough to feel a shift.

Trust me—if I can lose weight with tapping, and my clients can lose weight with tapping, you can, too!

# Chapter 3

# Ending the Pattern of Panic

Now that we've learned how stress negatively impacts the weight loss and body confidence journey and how tapping helps us overcome the damaging impacts of stress on weight and the body, we need to address the most common roadblock women encounter when they're beginning this journey: panic. Feeling panicked about the need to lose weight and feel good can take many forms and be triggered by a variety of circumstances.

## The Pattern of Panic

"I feel like I need to lose 50 to 80 pounds in the next three weeks," Analisa wrote. In a few weeks' time she would be seeing a friend she hadn't seen since she'd gained the weight. She was sure her friend would see her as nothing more than "fat," and she couldn't stop playing an imaginary movie in her head—her friend calling their mutual friends to tell them how fat she'd become. Overwhelmed by fear and anxiety, she wanted nothing more than to fend off the silent ridicule she was sure her friend would pile on her.

Analisa was in a panic. For me, the panic to lose weight and feel good in my body began when I was 14, always while facing my then archenemy, the mirror, which never failed to display my body's so-called flaws. By my early 20s, the slightest glance at my reflection was enough to turn me into a drill sergeant. I would pinch and prod every inch of my body to prove my point—that I wasn't good enough.

The panic would hit me like a shot of adrenaline, and in a flash I'd be on the latest diet, dragging myself to the gym to try some new class. Nearly every time, I lost the weight—and then gained it all back. It was a pattern I couldn't seem to stop, but each time, I returned to my brutal but familiar old friend, panic. I worked myself up to playing the part of the drill sergeant, and then tore myself down until I couldn't help but dissolve into a puddle of desperate tears. I was never skinny enough, which to me meant I wasn't good enough. I felt like a failure everyone could see.

Years later, I began to understand the role panic had played in my tortured relationship with my weight. When I was in the heat of the moment, panic seemed like the only thing potent enough to get me to deal with the reflection in the mirror. Each time, panic forced me into action, and each time, I ended up right where I started.

On some level I knew I was repeating a tired old pattern of short-lived weight loss, but surely, I told myself, if I worked hard enough, deprived myself often enough, I would arrive at lifelong thinness . . . wouldn't I? I just couldn't quiet that abusive voice in my head that seemed to think so.

Like so many women who struggle with weight, Analisa and I both got stuck in what I call the pattern of panic. However common it may be, it's a pattern we must break free of to achieve long-term body confidence and weight loss. First, however, we need to take a closer look at what it is and why it happens.

## The Two Sides of Panic

Often when clients come to their first session with me, on the surface they seem to be having different experiences. Some seem ashamed that they need help losing weight, others are scared they'll be disappointed again, and still others seem prepared for some mild form of torture, ready and willing to do "whatever it takes." Beneath the surface, however, they're having very similar experiences. They're all stuck in the pattern of panic, convinced they need to shed the pounds now—*right* now.

We tend to react to the pattern of panic in one of two ways—fight or admit defeat. While these tactics may seem like polar opposites, they're both reactions to the underlying panic we're feeling about needing to lose the weight and feel confident in our own skin. Some of us tend toward one reaction while others vacillate between the two reactions over time.

## THE "FIGHT" PATTERN OF PANIC

The "fight" reaction to panic around losing weight often comes on very suddenly, triggered by a specific memory or event, like Analisa's realization that her friend's visit was only three weeks away. In the fight reaction, we're overwhelmed by a feeling of desperation to lose the weight now at (almost) any cost. In those moments we're convinced that weight is the full measure of our value as individuals. Nothing else about who we are, what we have to offer, or what we've accomplished can possibly have as much worth as our weight.

That's what happened to Analisa. Overcome by shame, fear, and anxiety, she couldn't imagine enjoying her visit with her friend; all she could do was feel threatened by it. The story running through her head was the only outcome she could envision. Every time Analisa thought about meeting her friend, she was preparing herself mentally and emotionally to fend off the backstabbing, judgmental attack that seemed inevitable.

When we're experiencing this fight reaction, we tell ourselves that we need the panic—no matter how painful it is—because panic is our last hope. If we stop panicking, we are giving up on losing the weight. We believe that we *have* to be hard on ourselves because when we're not, we gain the weight back. The panic itself becomes a reason to believe that we can still somehow lose the weight.

## THE "DEFEAT" PATTERN OF PANIC

Compared to the fight reaction to panic, the "defeat" pattern of panic can seem deceptively calm.

"It's my badge of failure," Joni said of her weight. The worst part, she added, was that everyone could see her badge of failure, every single day.

"How much motivation do you feel to take care of your body when you see it as your badge of failure?" I asked.

"None," she replied.

"I don't blame you," I told her. "If I saw my body as a badge of failure, I wouldn't take care of it, either. Who would want to spend time caring for something they hate?"

At first glance the defeat pattern can seem like the exact opposite of panic. It looks like giving up, like we don't care about our weight. Junk food, overeating, not exercising—all the ways we abuse ourselves and our bodies seem justified. We have gained the weight and failed to lose it. We have been deeply disappointed by our failure to lose the weight. We have spent so much energy fighting; enough is enough. Finally, we are waving the white flag, admitting defeat. It's the smart thing to do, we tell ourselves. The weight loss programs and diets that everyone else lost weight on don't work for us. Being fat is who we are, so why fight what we clearly can't control?

Below the surface, however, we never do accept our weight. We cannot. We think about our weight constantly but we can't face the disappointment and pain behind it—not again. It's too overwhelming, too deep. It would break us. Instead, we wear defeat like a mask, a disguise to cover the shame and self-blame we stuff ourselves with. Beneath the surface, we're just as panicked about our weight as when we are in fight mode. In fact, in the defeat pattern of panic, we may feel more desperate and anxious than ever.

# Why We Panic

When we're panicked about weight, whether we're having a fight or defeat reaction, we feel sure that losing all the weight will fix everything. In panic mode, even when we appear to have given up, nothing seems as important to us as losing the weight. If we could only lose the weight, we tell ourselves, everything would be different, our lives would be different, *we* would be different.

Our panic begins to feel more powerful than we are, so we buy into the idea mass media and mass culture sell us every day—that thin equals happy and carefree. If or when I lose the weight, we each tell ourselves, my relationships will improve, my career will take off, my house will finally be neat and clean. When we lose the weight, life will just *work*. The possibility that life could just work at our current weight doesn't compute.

To anyone who hasn't gone through this pattern of panic around weight loss, the experience may sound insane. In many ways it is. When we're in it, however, nothing feels more legitimate. We're under a dangerous spell but we can't yet see that, so off we go to buy another diet book or try the newest way to exercise; or off we go on another downward spiral, diving into another box of treats because there is no more hope that we can lose the weight.

On some level, of course, we know that panic isn't delivering the long-term weight loss we want, but time and time again we return to it. Why is that? What's our panic really about?

*The panic comes because we want to avoid and deny what we don't want to talk about—that our struggle with weight isn't actually about the weight. When we panic about losing weight, what we're dying for is to be ourselves.* We want to feel like we are okay just as we are. We panic because it's all consuming, because it allows us to ignore something that feels too painful to admit: that we don't actually believe that we are enough; that we've gotten very comfortable with denying our own worth. But our weight, of course, isn't the sum total of our worth. It is, however, a crutch. We tell ourselves that once we "fix" ourselves by losing the weight, we will finally be worthy of happiness, love, suc-cess—anything and everything that seems to be missing in our lives.

Over and over again, we're seduced by this idea that our panic may someday bring us sustainable weight loss and, therefore, happiness. The truth is, however, that we can be happy at any weight if we value ourselves.

## Breaking the Pattern of Panic

Like many of my clients, you may be terrified to stop panicking because you equate not panicking with accepting that you'll never lose weight. But you also know that panic isn't the answer. If panic worked, you'd have lost the weight for good. If panic helped, you wouldn't be read-ing this book.

It's time to stop the pattern of panic once and for all. It's time to admit that your weight loss isn't about your weight. The fact is that until you lower your stress and clear your emotional residue and nega-tive beliefs, sustainable weight loss will seem out of your reach. You will hear me say this often, but here's the truth: long-term weight loss and body confidence is an inside job.

For Analisa, that journey began with tapping around her panic about her friend's visit. After calming her panic, she realized that her fears were unfounded. She was vastly underestimating both her friend and the friendship she and this person had. She had always been good at picking friends, and this person would never judge her so harshly for her weight. In fact, she realized that she was projecting onto her friend how cruel she often was to herself.

When they did finally meet, she was able to be present with her friend and really bond with her. Throughout their time together, she laughed and had a truly great time. That was a big shift com-pared to the previous time she had seen old friends and felt emo-tionally guarded and uncomfortable in her body. During this visit, Analisa could clearly see that her weight didn't have to interfere with her reunion. Her friend wanted to catch up with Analisa, not

Analisa-at-a-certain-weight. It makes you think: *How often have I robbed myself of an incredible experience because of my own internal fears and judgments around my body?*

Analisa's story is just one example of the ways in which the pattern of panic prevents us from looking at how we may be projecting our poor self-image onto others and denying the underlying issues that prevent us from experiencing sustainable weight loss. It's time to end the pattern of panic. But before we do tapping to begin quieting the panic, we need to address the two most common triggers of weight loss panic—the mirror and the scale.

## Panic Trigger #1: The Mirror

Cindy walked into her closet with little time to spare before party guests would begin arriving. The Fourth of July party she and her husband hosted each year was about to begin, and she only had a few minutes to change. As she looked in her closet, she reminded herself that her husband's entire family would once again be coming. They'd seen her gain and lose weight several times during their ten-year marriage, and each year she felt ashamed that they had witnessed the outward results of this very private struggle.

> You've been criticizing yourself for years and it hasn't worked.
> Try approving of yourself and see what happens.
>
> —LOUISE L. HAY

Before last year's party, in fact, she had locked herself in her room, showered, and tried on dozens of outfits, only to end up sobbing on the floor of her closet. All she could think of was that people would look at her and think she was fat. She felt panicked and depressed, unsure whether she could face her own family and friends.

This year, however, Cindy had come prepared. She had bought a beautiful new dress just for the occasion. She quickly put it on and turned toward the mirror. She immediately began inspecting every angle of her reflection, telling herself once again that she looked fat and that everyone would notice and talk about how fat she was.

Because Cindy had just begun my class, things were different this year. She paused long enough to notice her critical thoughts about herself. With only a few minutes to spare, she did some tapping. While looking at herself in the mirror and tapping, she then did something she rarely does. She looked at herself and said out loud, "You look beautiful."

Smiling and feeling relaxed, she opened the door to her room and went to join the party. Throughout the day, and for the first time ever, Cindy didn't think about whether she looked fat. She didn't obsess about food. Instead she enjoyed feeling peaceful and calm. Through-out the day, people showered her with compliments, telling her how pretty she looked. What surprised her more was how pretty she *felt*.

What's so inspiring to me about Cindy's story is that she was able to change her entire day just by noticing her negative thoughts and self-talk. She could then tap and accept a positive belief instead—that she looked beautiful. Rather than spending the entire party thinking about her looks, she radiated beauty, and of course, everyone noticed! She also shared that she was surprised to find she was feeling so good and having so much fun that she didn't feel her usual stress around food at parties. The panic of "should I or shouldn't I eat this" disap-peared, and she found herself enjoying healthier options.

So many of my clients have experienced powerful shifts in their emotional state and self-perception while tapping in front of the mirror. Often at first, it's scary facing your reflection while tapping. The mirror has become your nemesis, the enemy that exposes your most humiliat-ing flaws. Faced with your own reflection, you examine your every inch, top to bottom, front to back, side to side. Frantically but methodically, you point out every last lump and bump. You give yourself no mercy and think and say things you would never say to those you love.

I have worked with women who wake up, run to the mirror, and begin measuring themselves up and down to decide whether they'll have a good day. I've also worked with women who shower in the dark to avoid the mirror, knowing it will instantaneously dampen their mood. We give the mirror, a piece of glass, the power to dictate our happiness, not because we're vain but because we haven't invested in our relationship with ourselves or the body we currently have. What we see in the mirror is a reflection of our relationship with ourselves, and all too often that relationship is suffering from years of neglect.

Let's take a closer look at how you're treating that woman in the mirror. As you inspect every inch of your reflection, you may find that you shower yourself with deeply hurtful words that would make you outraged if you heard them said to anyone else. You know that the people you love can't thrive under constant scrutiny, yet you may discover that you punish yourself in this way endlessly. The first step in beginning to repair your relationship with yourself is awareness.

## WHAT'S YOUR RELATIONSHIP WITH THE MIRROR?

Take a moment now to ask yourself these questions:

- What is my relationship to the mirror?
- Do I avoid it?
- Do I spend a long time in front of it critiquing myself?

Notice what you say to yourself when you're faced with your own reflection and write those words down.

Whatever your answers, when you approach the mirror you will find what you're looking for. If you're looking for flaws you will find them. If you're looking for things to appreciate, you'll find those. You may think that you need the critique and that by being hard on yourself, you will be shielded from other people's judgments about you. In fact, as we saw with Cindy, when you appreciate yourself and your own beauty, you radiate that beauty to everyone around you.

As you look at yourself, notice any critical self-talk or emotions that surface. If an emotion comes up, measure it on a scale of 0 to 10 and write it down. The key here is to give that emotion or critical self-talk a voice as you tap. The tapping script below may serve as a guide to get you started. Do a few rounds of tapping and check in to see how you feel. You may find that the intensity increases when you begin tapping; this may simply be because this is the first time you've given a voice to these words you say to yourself on a regular basis. This is a sign that you've hit the nail on the head, so keep tapping!

**Karate Chop:** Even though I feel panic as I harshly judge the image in the mirror, I love and accept myself. *(Repeat this three times.)*

**Eyebrow:** Noticing everything I don't like . . .

**Side of Eye:** I'm standing in front of my harshest critic.

**Under Eye:** There is no way to feel happy with this image.

**Under Nose:** How did I let myself get like this?

**Chin:** All these emotions I face in front of the mirror . . .

**Collarbone:** I allow myself to give them a voice.

**Under Arm:** This feeling of panic . . .

**Top of Head:** Rejecting the person in the mirror.

*The key is to give a conscious voice to the words you would say to your reflection in the mirror as you do the tapping. When you feel like you can say those words without feeling like they are completely true, move on to the positive. This is all part of the same tapping sequence, so there's no need for another Karate Chop setup statement.*

**Eyebrow:** I have been so hard on you.

**Side of Eye:** You deserve more than this.

**Under Eye:** You don't need to do anything to deserve love.

**Under Nose:** I love you now.

**Chin:** I choose to appreciate you for all you do.

## Why We Tap on the Negative Before the Positive

Although we may have every intention of being kinder to ourselves, it often feels impossible because our negative words feel so true. When we feel panic in our bodies, it's hard to simply change our mind. When we tap on how we feel first, we can feel calm even when those negative thoughts come up. Then, once we're feeling more relaxed, we can move on to something more empowering.

**Collarbone:** I choose to speak kindly to you.

**Under Arm:** I love you, body.

**Top of Head:** I promise to take steps to express all the love you deserve.

*Take a deep breath and check in with how you feel. Measure the intensity again and continue tapping until you experience relief. For an extended tapping script on this topic, go to www.TheTappingSolution.com/chapter3.*

## Panic Trigger #2: The Scale

During the first session of my online weight loss class, I tell my students that they can weigh themselves once at the start of the class if they want to, and then they should put the scale away. Without fail, in session after session, women continue to obsess about the number they saw on the scale that morning. They report their results like you would confess your sins to a priest, subtly shaming themselves for not meeting their expectations.

Over and over again throughout the class, women talk about how their clothes feel looser and how they physically feel lighter. Just when

> Calm and confident isn't
> a number on the scale.
>
> —JESSICA ORTNER

I'm about to congratulate them, they share how depressed they feel because when they stepped on the scale this morning, their weight didn't reflect the big shift they feel. Maybe they gained a pound, stayed the same, or only lost a few pounds. They see the number and feel disappointed. Ugh. How did the scale become our private addiction?

To give us some perspective on how the scale became such an important way to measure our bodies, it's interesting to look at the history of the scale itself. The first one arrived in the United States from Germany in 1885. It wasn't until the 1920s and 1930s, however, that the scale was introduced to the general public. Massive machines weighing in at 200 pounds each, scales began to appear on street corners and in department stores, movie theaters, and public restrooms. They soon became a highly lucrative business, costing consumers a penny per weigh and producing millions in profit per year, even during the Great Depression of the 1930s.

To get a sense of how drastically our relationship to the scale has changed since then, imagine yourself willingly stepping on a scale in public, with dozens of strangers looking on. For most of us, that's a living nightmare. Weighing ourselves became a private event in the 1940s when technology advances paved the way for the manufacture of smaller, in-home scales.

Since then, mass culture has slowly but surely brainwashed us into believing that thin means beautiful, happy, worthy, confident, capable, lovable, and successful. As a result, the number we see on the scale has gone from an interesting curiosity to a judgment on our value as women. We know on some deeper level that our worth extends beyond what we weigh, but we continue to place more importance on the number we see on the scale than on how we feel in our own bodies. How can we break this pattern?

First, let's discuss the biggest myth about weight—the idea that your weight shouldn't fluctuate. Biologically speaking, that idea has zero merit, especially for women. As your hormones fluctuate so does your weight, not just during your menstrual cycle but also when your stress level increases. That fluctuation is a natural and healthy process, not something you need to "fix."

When we add in lifestyle factors and the effects of stress, the daily and weekly fluctuations you see on the scale become even more understandable. Here's a partial list of factors that can cause the number on the scale to go up and down, from hour to hour, day to day, and week to week:

| | | | |
|---|---|---|---|
| Changes in diet | Eating foods you're allergic to | Medications | Travel |
| Constipation | | Menstrual cycle | When you last ate |
| Dieting | Exercise | Sleep | |
| Eating close to bedtime | How much water you do or don't drink | Stress | When you last drank water or any beverage |
| | | Supplements | |

What's interesting is that the normal and healthy fluctuations in your weight don't always occur in ways you would expect. For instance, as we've seen, when your stress levels rise, your levels of cortisol also rise. In excessive amounts cortisol can cause your body to retain water. Because dieting puts your body under stress, when you first begin a diet your cortisol levels rise, which may cause your body to retain extra water. So when you step on the scale in those early days or weeks of a diet, it may look like you've gained weight!

The same principle can apply to changes in the way you eat. If you begin gravitating toward vegetables and fruits more than you have in the past, your body will notice a difference and may initially retain water; it's adjusting to these very positive changes in your eating and simultaneously preparing to lose weight.

I share all of this not so you obsess about what's affecting the number on the scale but so we can have a more informed discussion about why the scale is such a misleading and self-destructive way to track weight loss. In so many ways the number we see when we step on the scale is meaningless. To break our addiction to the scale, we need to first understand that, and then talk about why it's so hard for us to trust how our bodies feel. When clients say they feel lighter and their clothes are fitting better, why do they still insist on stepping on the scale?

## RELEARNING HOW TO TRUST YOUR BODY

During our years of losing and gaining weight, many of us have come to mistrust our bodies. We've spent years resisting the body's natural urges to eat and experience pleasure, and then we've tortured ourselves with guilt and shame when we give in to these positive and healthy urges. Over time, the bodies we live in become enemies conspiring to make us gain weight rather than things we love, respect, and care for. Given this mistrust we feel, our reliance on the scale as proof of our weight loss (or not) makes perfect sense. After all, how can we trust the way the body feels when it has been working against us for so long?

> Our inner guidance comes to us first through our feelings and body wisdom—not through intellectual understanding.
>
> —CHRISTIANE NORTHRUP, M.D.

The scale, like the mirror, quickly becomes a sort of dictator. Based on whatever number appears, the scale tells you whether you're allowed to have a good day, whether you're allowed to feel happy, beautiful, and worthy. The problem is that not trusting your body and punishing yourself for a "bad" number ultimately make it harder, not easier, to lose the weight. Because you can't trust your own body, you may feel stressed when you don't step on the scale or when the number on the scale isn't what you're hoping for.

One of my students, Robyn, had a breakthrough about the usefulness of the scale in her own weight loss journey a few weeks into my online class:

> Since week 1, I have thought about your "hide your scale" directive. I immediately liked the idea because I knew that if I was

making some effort (in this case, tapping) and not getting results (the number on the scale going down), then I would be adding unnecessary emotional baggage to the pile of issues I already know I need to deal with around my weight and body.

This morning, I realized that NOT weighing myself is a better way to keep me accountable. By not weighing myself, I am supporting myself. I am holding myself accountable to my commitment to this class and to my own weight loss, and I have to say, it feels empowering. I love the feeling of doing something different! For once, I am not using my weight as a punishment but instead am freeing myself to actually do something good for me.

The scale is just a machine that's designed to give you a very basic piece of information—what you weigh at one specific moment in time. It isn't a judgment and it doesn't predict what you will weigh tomorrow, next week, or next month. To begin ingraining that idea into your brain, let's now do some tapping around your relationship with the scale and around relearning how to trust your body.

**Karate Chop:** Even though I've allowed the scale to measure my worth, I love and accept myself and choose to take my power back. (*Repeat three times.*)

**Eyebrow:** I can't stop looking at the number.

**Side of Eye:** It tells me how I should feel.

**Under Eye:** It tells me if I'm being good or bad.

**Under Nose:** I've lost trust in myself.

**Chin:** So I trust in this scale . . .

**Collarbone:** To tell me how I'm doing.

**Under Arm:** I have to look at the scale.

**Top of Head:** That's the only way to know I'm "good."

*Continue tapping and even exaggerate your beliefs about the scale until they don't feel true. Then move on to the positive.*

**Eyebrow:** I choose to take my power back.

**Side of Eye:** Instead of checking in with the scale . . .

**Under Eye:** I check in with myself.

**Under Nose:** I'm aware of how my body feels.

**Chin:** And I know what my body really needs.

**Collarbone:** Calm and confident isn't a number on the scale.

**Under Arm:** It's who I am right now.

**Top of Head:** I choose to check in with myself instead of the scale.

*Take a deep breath and check in with how you feel. Measure the intensity again and continue tapping until you experience relief.*

## The Power of Patience

When we get trapped in the pattern of panic, that's a sign that we need to find ways to love and accept ourselves in the moment. By doing that, we can experience more joy in our daily lives, and as a result be more patient with the process of losing weight in a healthy and sustainable way. When we fall in love with the journey, we can more easily move toward our dreams and celebrate every step forward. Luckily, time flies when you're having fun.

The true power of patience became clear to Gail early in her weight loss and body confidence journey. Having dreamt about wearing dresses for many years, she had always told herself that she would wear dresses when she could fit into a smaller size. While stuffing herself with food that didn't make her body feel good, Gail was unconsciously depriving herself of a simple but important pleasure—the experience of wearing clothes that made her feel pretty.

A couple of weeks into my class, Gail shared some exciting news. She had bought herself several new dresses and now wore them often. They made her feel feminine, confident, and beautiful, and for the first time in many years, she didn't hate her own reflection in the mirror.

Since beginning to look at the underlying issues of her struggle with weight and using tapping to clear her resistance to taking care of herself, Gail felt empowered around food. Without feeling deprived, she found herself choosing healthy, nourishing foods, eating less, and thinking about food less as well. The class had barely begun, and already Gail was getting incredible results—results that I knew would soon translate into noticeable weight loss.

Gail is one of thousands of students who have reaffirmed what I myself experienced—when weight loss becomes a pleasurable experience, we achieve the weight loss we desire, and so much more. Too many of us, like Gail, have made weight loss into the dream that must come before all others. We tell ourselves that until we lose the weight we can't fall in love or start a new career. Until we lose the weight, we can't appreciate ourselves, enjoy our lives, or wear clothes that make us feel beautiful. Because of weight, we put our lives on hold, often letting months and years pass us by.

When we can quiet the panic and practice patience with the weight loss journey, we open ourselves to the possibilities of the present. We begin to see that our lives can be amazing, inspiring, and pleasurable, not just after we lose the weight but now—*right now*. When we can enjoy the adventure, we arrive at the destination so much faster than we ever imagined and we have a blast doing it. This is the power of patience, and this is what I want for you, starting right now and continuing throughout your journey.

Once you've begun to quiet the panic, you're ready for the next phase of the journey. Part II, which begins with Chapter 4, will help you learn about yourself; it will help you peel the onion and address any long-standing obstacles that have been preventing you from losing weight or feeling confident in your body. But first it's time to do some tapping to unleash the power of patience for you, in your own journey of weight loss and body confidence.

# Experiencing the Power of Patience

**Karate Chop:** Even though I can't relax until I lose the weight, I love and accept myself. (*Repeat three times.*)

**Eyebrow:** This panic . . .

**Side of Eye:** The need to punish myself . . .

**Under Eye:** The weight of this weight . . .

**Under Nose:** This pressure in my body . . .

**Chin:** This pressure I put on myself . . .

**Collarbone:** I feel the need to criticize myself . . .

**Under Arm:** To judge myself.

**Top of Head:** I can't accept myself when I look like this.

**Eyebrow:** All of this pressure . . .

**Side of Eye:** It's hard to think of anything else.

**Under Eye:** My life feels like it's on hold.

**Under Nose:** I can't be happy until I lose this weight.

**Chin:** I can't feel confident until I lose the weight.

**Collarbone:** I can't enjoy the moment until I lose the weight.

**Under Arm:** No wonder I panic about my weight . . .

**Top of Head:** I allow it to stop me from living life.

**Eyebrow:** I feel I need to criticize myself . . .

**Side of Eye:** So that I finally change.

**Under Eye:** But this approach hasn't been working . . .

**Under Nose:** I would never speak to someone I love like this.

**Chin:** All of this judgment and body shaming . . .

**Collarbone:** Is keeping me stuck.

**Under Arm:** This emotional weight I carry with the weight . . .

**Top of Head:** I'm ready to let go of this emotional weight now.

**Eyebrow:** Maybe the weight isn't holding me back.

**Side of Eye:** I've been holding myself back.

**Under Eye:** I no longer wait for the weight . . .

**Under Nose:** I honor myself now . . .

**Chin:** From this space anything is possible.

**Collarbone:** I make choices that empower me.

**Under Arm:** I create a loving internal environment for my body.

**Top of Head:** It's been so good under these hard circumstances.

**Eyebrow:** I appreciate my body with loving words.

**Side of Eye:** Thank you for all you do for me.

**Under Eye:** You don't need to earn my love.

**Under Nose:** I love you now, as you are.

**Chin:** You've been so good to me . . .

**Collarbone:** I continue to discover ways to take care of you . . .

**Under Arm:** With loving words and actions.

**Top of Head:** I choose to feel the love I have for you.

**Eyebrow:** Instead of checking in with the mirror . . .

**Side of Eye:** Or the scale . . .

**Under Eye:** I check in with myself . . .

**Under Nose:** And give myself the care I deserve.

**Chin:** I trust in this process.

**Collarbone:** I trust in life.

**Under Arm:** It's all unfolding as it should.

**Top of Head:** I enjoy this moment.

# Part II

# Looking Within

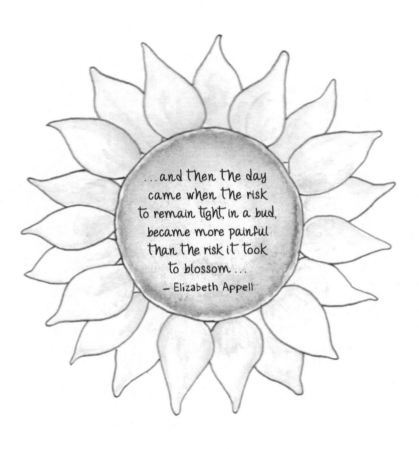

...and then the day came when the risk to remain tight, in a bud, became more painful than the risk it took to blossom ...
— Elizabeth Appell

# Chapter 4

# Overcoming Emotional Eating

Emotional eating often feels like our own dirty little secret, the source of equal servings of pleasure and shame. When we're under the influence of emotional eating—whether we're indulging a food craving, overeating to avoid our emotions, or constantly snacking—food becomes a toxic love affair. One moment we're smitten, soothed in body and soul by whatever we're eating. The next thing we know, we're uncomfortably full, trying to digest equally oversized servings of food and guilt.

Making the final break from emotional eating can be incredibly difficult without tapping. It's a behavioral pattern that we often don't believe we can control. When we feel emotionally vulnerable, it's easy to crawl back into the arms of food. It never judges you. It's always there to comfort you. Food makes you feel happy and free until the toxic cycle of overindulgence and guilt repeats itself.

Next we'll explore the different forms of emotional eating and then discover how to break free from emotional eating. First, however, we need to understand more about this misunderstood topic by looking at why we tend to overindulge in certain kinds of foods.

# Why We Overeat

When we're taking a closer look at emotional eating behaviors, it's important to consider how the food we turn to when we're under the influence of emotional eating impacts our physiology. Most of us tend to indulge in simple carbohydrates—sugary or salty high-carbohydrate foods like cookies, chips, candy, ice cream, and more. What's interesting is that these foods can act like drugs in the body, making us feel calm and happy very quickly, although only for a short time.

> Self-sabotage is simply misguided self-love.
>
> —BRAD YATES

Science has confirmed that simple carbohydrates increase the concentration of an amino acid called tryptophan in the brain. Tryptophan is a building block of serotonin, a transmitter that, when released, gives you that calm, happy feeling. In other words, part of the reason it's so difficult to put the bag of chips or box of sweet treats down is that while you eat these foods, your brain is "high" on serotonin. The foods themselves trigger the reward centers in your brain, flooding your system with "feel good" chemicals. For a brief time, you feel amazing. It's no wonder you struggle to stop after just one cookie!

During an interview I did with tapping expert Brad Yates, he said something that struck me: "Self-sabotage is simply misguided self-love." When I began thinking about how that applies to emotional eating, I could see exactly how true that statement felt.

When we're in that moment of serotonin-fueled bliss, emotional eating feels like a way to nurture, love, and validate ourselves. We may think something like, *I did so much today, I deserve this*. Using food as a reward isn't a habit we picked up by ourselves. Thinking back to childhood, how many times were we told that if we were good we'd get a cookie? In that moment we understood that sugary treats are a way to appreciate our own goodness. It makes perfect sense, then, that in adulthood we continue to see food as a way to reward ourselves.

# Food Cravings: When the I NEED IT NOW! Urge Strikes

Succumbing to cravings is an incredibly common form of emotional eating, even though at the moment when the craving strikes, it often feels like a very real physical need. Cravings are also a symptom we experience in our struggle with weight loss.

Jenna experienced such intense cravings for her favorite snack, Ritz crackers with cream cheese, that she found herself driving faster on her way home from work in anticipation of eating them. Once home, she dove into her favorite treat before even closing the cupboard door. Then she zoned out, eating past the point of fullness while standing in front of the kitchen counter. It was a bad habit, she knew, but she couldn't seem to stop it.

One day Jenna did some tapping on her craving while driving home, taking a moment to tap at every red light. Once she got home, she felt so relaxed and in control that she didn't feel the need to rush into the kitchen. Her physical craving wasn't hijacking her anymore. She later realized that what she had really been craving was a way to let go of the workday, and simply tapping on the symptom—the craving—had taken care of this desire to eat.

This "symptom tapping," which is tapping on the craving itself, can often produce very fast results.

To begin addressing cravings you may have, let's now do some tapping directly on the food you most often crave. Just by tapping on the craving itself and the feeling of desperation around needing it, you can calm the body and relieve the craving.

Really think about the food you're craving; even try to intensify the craving. Give your craving a number of intensity from 0 to 10 and begin tapping while you focus on that craving sensation. Here is an example:

**Karate Chop:** Even though I need this chocolate, I accept how I feel and it's safe to relax now. (*Repeat three times.*)

**Eyebrow:** I need this chocolate.

**Side of Eye:** I have to have it now.

**Under Eye:** This craving for chocolate . . .

**Under Nose:** This pressure in my body . . .

**Chin:** I need it now.

**Collarbone:** This craving for chocolate . . .

**Under Arm:** This intense craving . . .

**Top of Head:** I can't focus on anything else.

*Check in with yourself. Has the intensity of your craving shifted? Continue tapping until the intensity is 5 or lower before moving to the positive round.*

**Eyebrow:** I can have the chocolate . . .

**Side of Eye:** Or not have the chocolate.

**Under Eye:** I feel calm now.

**Under Nose:** I feel centered now.

**Chin:** Maybe I'll have some now.

**Collarbone:** Maybe I'll have some later.

**Under Arm:** I am in control.

**Top of Head:** I choose what's best for me.

*Take a deep breath and check in with how you feel. Measure the intensity again and continue tapping until you experience relief.*

When cravings strike and feel too strong to resist, you can tap on them first thing each morning. That calming effect will help you throughout the day.

# When the Craving Won't Go Away

While most food cravings are tied to emotions, some are more deeply rooted in emotions than others. When symptom tapping doesn't calm your desire to indulge, that's usually a sign that your craving is tied to deeper emotions. In the moment, however, it may not seem like you're having a deep emotional experience. More likely it feels like the cookies are screaming, "*Eat me now!*" That's because your body is stuck in a panic response, making it impossible to reason your way through the experience. To figure out the real source of your craving, you first need to do some tapping to quiet the panic. You might begin by tapping on your karate chop point with a setup statement like, "Even though I can't get rid of this craving for cookies, I love and accept myself, and I'm okay."

Once you've done some tapping to quiet that initial panic and connect to your intuition, you may find it easier to answer the question, "What am I *really* craving?" This is when things get fun. You become your own investigator, able to tap on the emotions that are fueling your emotional eating.

Before doing some investigating of our own, let's discuss what's happening behind the scenes, in our unconscious mind, when we resort to emotional eating behaviors, including food cravings. The unconscious mind, which includes the almond-shaped amygdala in the brain, is charged with keeping us safe. It's designed to protect us from emotions, experiences, and memories that seem threatening. In this way emotional eating becomes useful, because while we're inhaling an entire pizza or chocolate cake, we're better able to avoid facing whatever experiences, memories, or emotions the unconscious mind has labeled as threatening.

When we get clear on what we're really craving—the unmet need the unconscious mind is using emotional eating to avoid—we can fill that need with a healthier habit. That's when real and lasting change occurs, as it did for Jenna, who realized she could use tapping to lower her stress after work instead of stuffing herself with Ritz crackers and cream cheese.

From one person to the next, sometimes one day to the next, there is a broad range of emotions that the unconscious mind may be trying

## Cravings Are Rarely Just about the Food

As you continue tapping on your stress, you may experience a shift in your cravings even when you don't focus on them directly. That's what happened to Sarah. A couple of weeks into my class, without ever tapping on her daily craving for sugary soda, she lost the desire to drink it. That's often a benefit of tapping. As we begin to clear the underlying issues that lead us toward emotional eating, we no longer need the numbing effect that food has given us. As a result, we naturally move away from the foods we once craved.

to avoid, using emotional eating as a convenient distraction. While it can be an intense emotion such as anger, there is no hard-and-fast rule. One emotion we tend to underestimate is boredom, a common source of emotional eating. Rather than signaling that you need a new activity or diversion, persistent boredom can be an indication that there's a lack of passion in your life. That unmet need for passion can lead you to seek pleasure in food, which provides a temporary "high."

For a more complete list of the feelings you may be trying to avoid through emotional eating, you may want to refer back to the more comprehensive list of emotions that tapping can clear in Chapter 2 (page 30).

## Discovering the Root of Your Emotional Eating

Now that we've discussed what emotional eating is and why it's so hard to stop without tapping, it's time to return to investigative work and figure out what's fueling your emotional eating.

## WHEN EMOTIONAL EATING IS A
## WAY TO AVOID CERTAIN FEELINGS

When we feel like we're dying to devour the nearest treat, we're often trying to avoid challenging emotions. That was the case for Joanne, who realized by tapping on her cravings how often she had been using food to "stuff down" her feelings. It wasn't just one or two specific emotions that she was trying to avoid, but the actual experience of feeling her emotions *at all* that frequently sent her running to the kitchen.

> Your appetite is designed like an airplane instrument panel—to warn you when spiritual and emotional fuel runs low. Hunger is a flashing red light signaling, "I need more peace of mind."
>
> — DOREEN VIRTUE

Samantha, on the other hand, realized one day that she had been resorting to emotional eating to avoid a specific feeling. A retired teacher and aspiring author, she had spent all morning working on her children's book but had made very little progress. When lunchtime rolled around, she went into her kitchen intending to make a healthy lunch. The moment she spotted the two boxes of cookies in her cabinet, however, she felt desperate to devour them all.

As soon as her craving hit, she began tapping while standing in her kitchen and realized that an old fear-fueled "tape" had been running through her brain. The tape was her mind's way of expressing her fear and anxiety around her book. It went something like this: *I'll never get published . . . who am I to write this book, anyway? I'm not a real writer.* Once she had tapped on her fear and anxiety around writing, her craving for cookies vanished and she was able to enjoy a healthy and satisfying lunch.

## WHAT FEELING(S) ARE YOU TRYING TO AVOID
## THROUGH EMOTIONAL EATING BEHAVIORS?

Take a moment now to ask yourself what feeling(s) you are trying to avoid. Tapping while asking yourself a question can calm your mind enough that it then becomes easier to access the answer. If you find it helpful to tap through the points each time you ask yourself a question during the exercises, feel free to do that for each of them.

Here's a tapping script to get you started:

**Karate Chop:** Even though I need this food to quiet this feeling, I love and accept myself. (*Repeat three times.*)

**Eyebrow:** I need to eat this now.

**Side of Eye:** I feel this feeling building up.

**Under Eye:** I don't want to feel it.

**Under Nose:** It's too much to handle.

**Chin:** It feels hopeless . . .

**Collarbone:** So I need this food.

**Under Arm:** It's the only way I'll get through the day.

**Top of Head:** All of these feelings behind the craving . . .

*Ask yourself again: What emotions might be behind my emotional eating, whether it's overeating or indulging a craving? What emotions or negative thoughts am I trying to avoid? Get clear on these and write down their intensity on a scale of 0 to 10. Give those feelings a voice and continue tapping. Once you are at least below an intensity of 5, move on to the positive statements.*

**Eyebrow:** I feel the peace I crave.

**Side of Eye:** I feel the love I crave.

**Under Eye:** I don't need to find all the answers.

**Under Nose:** I simply find relief in this moment.

**Chin:** It's safe to feel these feelings . . .

**Collarbone:** And to let them go.

**Under Arm:** I can find the relaxation I crave now.

**Top of Head:** I honor my body by eating lovingly and consciously.

*Remember: as you do your tapping, use the tapping scripts I provide as your prompt and then move into your specific answer(s) to the question in each exercise.*

## Emotional Eating Triggers

Margaret had gained 15 pounds in six months. Feeling defeated and depressed, she shared that she couldn't stop snacking. "I work from home," she said, "and I find myself constantly in the kitchen. I can't figure out why." When I asked her what had happened six months earlier that would lead her to gain this weight, she said that was when she started her new job. "Is your new job stressful?" I asked. "Yes!" she blurted out. "My new boss is driving me crazy."

As we began tapping on the stress she was feeling because of her new boss, she began to see that grabbing a snack had become her way of taking a break. "I have such a hard time taking care of myself," she shared. "I try to be everything for everyone. I want to be a good mom. I want to be a successful career woman. I want to take care of my husband. There just isn't time for me. This new boss takes that pressure to a whole new level and it feels unbearable."

We also tapped on events that triggered her. We began tapping while she imitated all the things her boss said that made her panic. We continued tapping on those words until she could say them without feeling the familiar panic in her stomach. We were then able to bring in affirmations like "I am calm and centered in my body," "I know exactly what to do," and "I feel calm and confident." Then I had Margaret envision a clear bubble around her. While tapping through the points, I had her imagine that she could hear her boss's words but her boss's energy couldn't break the bubble. This process helped cement the idea that we can hear someone's words without taking on their panicked energy.

Before tapping, Margaret had felt that she needed to feel her boss's stress in order to be helpful at work. She had also equated being calm with not caring enough about her job. When she tapped, she realized she could hear her boss complain without picking up her boss's stress. By remaining calm and confident when her boss was stressed, Margaret could be more resourceful and helpful to her boss, not less.

General stress is a very common trigger for emotional eating, but there are also other, less expected triggers.

## THE REBELLION RESPONSE

It was just a few weeks into our work together, and Rebecca was feeling great. She had been tapping frequently and was enjoying eating healthier foods and exercising. Her energy and mood had been positive during our previous session, so I was concerned when she started this phone session with a panicked-sounding whisper.

"Are you okay?" I asked immediately.

"I'm visiting my dad but didn't want to cancel our session," she whispered.

She then shared that she had been eating terribly over the past couple of days and was feeling depressed about undoing her earlier progress. She believed it was just her lack of willpower and being around all the Fourth of July treats.

"Did something happen right before you found yourself emotionally eating?" I asked.

She paused and then said, "Oh, I know what it was."

Upon arriving at her dad's house, she had told him about the progress she'd been making while working with me. Instead of being excited for her, he had replied, "Oh, good—you could stand to lose some weight."

The comment had left Rebecca feeling hurt and alone, like she needed to lose weight in order to earn her dad's love. Like so many of my clients who struggle with weight, Rebecca's immediate reaction was to rebel against him. If he couldn't love her for who she was, her unconscious mind reasoned, then she would simply refuse to give in to his desires for her to lose weight. If he wanted to be her father, he would have to learn to love a "fat" Rebecca. Beneath her rebelliousness, however, Rebecca felt deeply wounded and was drowning in her own anger and sadness.

> When the world doesn't live up to our expectations, we rebel against its unfairness by turning to food.
>
> —JESSICA ORTNER

The urge to rebel against the pressure to lose weight often intersects with the weight loss journey. When the world doesn't live up to our expectations, we rebel against its unfairness by turning to food. Generally, emotional eating associated with this response comes immediately following an experience that triggers the subconscious belief about unfairness. In that moment, when we eat we feel like we're giving a middle finger to a society that is pressuring us into trying to live up to expectations that always seem beyond our reach. We give a middle finger to a father, mother, friend, or mentor who commented on our weight and made us feel like we could never be fully loved unless we lost weight and/or embodied the ideal they wanted to impose upon us.

When we're in rebellion, emotional eating is a way of giving ourselves that misguided self-love we talked about earlier. It's an immediate response that gives us the love others seem to be denying us. And for a brief time, it feels liberating—like we're taking back our power, taking charge when so much feels out of control. But in truth we are only waging a war on ourselves.

When you have this in-the-moment desire to eat, it is often sufficient to tap on the emotions the trigger brought up. However, if this doesn't relieve the desire, you sometimes have to go deeper and tap on the words or the event itself. We'll discuss just how to do this in the next chapter. For Rebecca this is exactly what happened. We began tapping on the anger behind her rebellion response, and soon she began remembering the many passive-aggressive comments her dad had made over the years about her weight, frequently pointing out thinner women and mentioning how good they looked. Over and over again, without ever blatantly criticizing her weight, he had made her feel less lovable and less worthy because of it. As we continued tapping through her emotions and memories, she was able to clear the enormous hurt and anger she had been keeping buried inside her. She knew that her journey to better health had nothing to do with her dad or social pressures; it was her personal journey to loving herself and seeing her own worth.

It was a huge relief for Rebecca to be able to let go of such a big emotional burden, and for the rest of her stay she was able to feel calm and eat in a manner that was both enjoyable and respectful to her body. What's even more interesting is that she had a better time with her father and could appreciate that he meant well, even if his actions and words felt hurtful.

For another one of my clients, we were able to stop her emotional eating simply by tapping on a feeling. Kristie, a working mom, realized through tapping that she was most often triggered to reach for food when she was exhausted. She calls it the "mommy munching" syndrome, because for her it began when her daughter was young. Every time she was able to take a break, such as when her daughter was napping, Kristie made food for herself, even when she wasn't hungry. Her habit of eating to relax became ingrained over time, perpetuating her struggle with weight. Once she was aware of this pattern, she was able to address her exhaustion more directly through tapping, opting for a nap, taking a hot bath, or exercising instead of eating.

The possible triggers for your emotional eating are nearly endless, so now let's figure out when you're triggered, and then do some tapping.


WHEN ARE YOU TRIGGERED TO ENGAGE
IN EMOTIONAL EATING?

Think about the last time you found yourself emotionally eating. Were you on the couch, standing over the kitchen counter, or in the car? Was it late at night or when you were alone in the house?

Get clear on that emotional eating event and then ask yourself, "Did something happen or did I have a particular feeling right before I began?" That answer gives you a tapping target, whether it's a feeling of exhaustion and frustration or something someone said or did. You can tap while giving a voice to that feeling.

## When Surrendering Emotional Eating Feels Like Self-Punishment

McDonald's and hot fudge sundaes were Tess's happy times. Never one to eat when she was upset, she turned to food when she was feeling good, excited to indulge in a pleasurable experience. Emotional eating, which for her was overeating, had been her main source of pleasure, a reward she deserved and didn't want to give up.

Like Tess, many of us become attached to emotional eating. It's a safety net, a reward, even a way to connect to the past—perhaps a reminder of the home-cooked meals Mom once so lovingly prepared. While we don't feel comfortable or happy when we're carrying excess weight, we resist the idea of giving up overeating because it has been our loyal companion for so long and the thought of giving it up feels unsafe.

Most of us aren't conscious of our relationship with overeating. It's important to stop and ask, "What's the downside of ending this habit?" This "downside" question is something we will visit many times throughout this book. In Tess's case, food was her way of celebrating her accomplishments, including surviving another day in a work environment that felt out of control. Without food, she wondered, how would she "treat" herself to feeling good?

A couple of weeks into my class, after taking moments throughout the day to tap on her stress, she experienced a drastic change. While riding in the car one day with her husband, just as they were nearing their favorite hot fudge sundae shop, he asked, "Are you going to ask me to pull over?"

Much to her shock (and his), she replied, "No, I don't really want it," with a smile.

Without the extra stress, she didn't need food to celebrate "surviving" another hard day. That same week, she found herself at the grocery store filling her basket with fresh produce and having no desire to walk down the cookie aisle. "It feels like my brain has been rewired,"

## Exploring "Secondary Gain"

Throughout the process of digging deeper into the underlying causes of our weight struggles, we'll be talking a lot about a crucial concept: "secondary gain." Secondary gain doesn't necessarily refer to weight; instead, it's a psychology term that refers to the secondary benefit of various conditions, such as illness, pain, and weight.

Years ago when I first began digging deeper into my own weight challenges, the possibility that I was holding on to weight for some reason kept occurring to me, but every time the thought crossed my mind I quickly found a reason to focus on something else. One day, however, I decided to ask myself two questions related to secondary gain that I'd learned from Carol Look, a tapping expert I'd interviewed for *The Tapping Solution* movie. The two questions were *"What's the benefit of holding on to weight?"* and conversely, *"What's the downside of losing weight?"* My initial answers were clear—"*nothing.*" For years I'd wanted nothing more than to *lose the weight.* Not being thin was *the* issue, *the* obstacle standing between me and happiness, me and success, me and my fabulous future.

As I continued tapping on these two questions, however, I had a major breakthrough. The floodgates opened and a stream of answers poured out of me. I was so stunned by what I'd discovered buried inside myself that I wrote the answers down. Here are some of them:

- If I'm successful at losing weight, I'll have to be on a restrictive diet.

- If I'm successful at losing weight, I'll be harshly judged by other women.

she said of how tapping has impacted her. Without feeling even a hint of deprivation, Tess is eating healthy food and enjoying it, able to reward herself in new and different ways that feel even more satisfying than sundaes.

- If I'm successful at losing weight, I'll be giving in to cultural pressures that I resent.

- If I lose the weight and pursue my dream and fail, it will mean something is wrong with me. I won't be able to blame the weight.

That breakthrough, which could not have happened without tapping, was the beginning of an entirely new relationship between me and my weight. As I continued tapping on all my resistance, I shed pounds faster and more easily than I ever had before and also began to feel lighter, more energetic, happier, and more confident in my own skin.

Like I once did, many of my students initially resist the opportunity to dig deeper into their weight and body stories but then have similarly significant breakthroughs as they look at the secondary gain of their own weight struggles.

While the process of digging deeper into your weight and body story may feel uncomfortable, even unsettling at times, I urge you to continue moving forward with this process. With tapping you don't need to go deep into the pain to find relief. You do, however, need to have the courage to take personal responsibility and face the parts of yourself and your life that you have been neglecting. You need to be willing to air out the parts of your life that are so desperate for attention that they are showing up as physical weight. With tapping, the process gets easier and is soon accompanied by positive physical and emotional changes.

# What's the Downside of Giving Up Emotional Eating?

Imagine that you couldn't overindulge in your favorite treat for a full week. Does that scenario create a sense of panic? What is the downside in ending this habit of emotional eating? Does a particular emotion or level of resistance come up? Write down your thoughts on a piece of paper, if you like, and use them as your tapping target. Remember to measure the intensity of your emotions before you begin tapping.

**Karate Chop:** Even though I'm unwilling to end this habit, I love and accept myself. (*Repeat three times.*)

**Eyebrow:** I don't want to stop craving this food.

**Side of Eye:** I don't want to deprive myself.

**Under Eye:** It's a way for me to avoid uncomfortable feelings.

**Under Nose:** It's a way to praise myself.

**Chin:** It's a way to experience pleasure.

**Collarbone:** I don't want to give it up.

**Under Arm:** I'm sick of this pressure.

**Top of Head:** I want to rebel and do what I want.

*Keep tapping on all the reasons you don't want to let go of this habit. When the intensity is 5 or lower, begin incorporating these positive tapping phrases.*

**Eyebrow:** I *can* do what I want.

**Side of Eye:** I can choose to eat whatever I want.

**Under Eye:** The calmer I feel . . .

**Under Nose:** The more control I have to choose what I really want.

**Chin:** I don't need the food in order to feel validated; I choose to feel validated now.

**Collarbone:** I don't need the food in order to feel calm; I choose to feel calm now.

**Under Arm:** It's safe for me to acknowledge what I really want.

**Top of Head:** I choose what I want from this calm and centered space.

*The point of this exercise isn't to prevent you from ever indulging in your favorite treat but simply to pinpoint the emotions that may be causing you to overindulge.*

Over time you may find these triggers reappearing or discover new emotional eating triggers. Don't let this discourage you. Simply take note of the triggers and then tap through them until they're fully cleared.

## What Are You Really Eating?

When emotional eating becomes a habit ingrained over many years, it can be hard to see all the ways in which our relationship with food is working against us. That became clear to me one evening while I was out with my friend and mentor Ariane de Bonvoisin, best-selling author of *The First 30 Days*. She had been raving about a gelato place in New York, claiming they had the best chocolate gelato in the entire city, so finally one night we went there to enjoy a treat.

After getting a serving each, we crossed the street to sit in a little plaza and enjoy our gelato. It was a beautiful summer evening, and for a moment we ate in silence, taking in the beauty of a nearby fountain.

Suddenly Ariane broke the silence. "You know we're eating two different things, don't you?"

I looked down at her cup. "No, I ordered the same thing as you."

"We are still eating two different things," she said. "I'm eating gelato—you're eating guilt. My body will enjoy and process this gelato perfectly and it will go right through me. That guilt will stick to you and you'll gain weight."

I was stunned into silence, shocked both by what she had said and how true it felt. I had been eating a healthy diet for some time but couldn't seem to lose weight. I suddenly realized that evening that the food group I had forgotten to cut out was guilt and shame.

Living in a culture that's obsessed with food and fitness, we're taught from a young age that carrying extra weight means that we're "less than," that we're overweight because we have no self-control. Deep down we know that's not true. We know we're amazing, inspiring, beautiful, and talented. And yet, through all of our years of struggling to lose the weight, we come to doubt ourselves. We come to downgrade our worth. Slowly but surely, we let our culture's fixation on thinness eat away at our self-confidence. Little by little, we put our own value into question. We feel ashamed of ourselves because our bodies don't meet our culture's strict and limiting standard of beauty. We wonder if we are actually flawed, when the real problem is that we haven't yet learned how to love and respect ourselves as we are. Food is not the enemy. It's time for us to end this cycle and stop inhaling a side of shame and guilt—and any other negative emotions—with each bite.

Take a moment now to think about how you feel when you eat. Ask yourself, *What emotions am I eating? Do I harshly judge myself and my worth when I eat?* As always, you may find the process easier if you do some tapping while thinking about and answering the questions.

## Let's Make Eating a Pleasurable Experience

Now that we've explored emotional eating in detail, I'd like to discuss an equally important topic: pleasure. While we'll explore the subject of self-care and pleasure in greater depth later in this journey, for the moment it's important to discuss the role pleasure plays in eating. What happens once we've used tapping to get rid of emotional eating behaviors? Are we left with nothing but wheatgrass and kale?

As you know, I don't believe in dieting. I believe in getting in tune with what your body needs and wants to feel great and be healthy. Again and again, I have seen that the weight naturally falls away once we've used tapping to clear the underlying issues around the relationship between ourselves and weight. At this point in the journey, however, when we think about eating healthier foods without doing the tapping around stress and the other underlying causes of emotional eating, we often equate healthy eating with deprivation. That's not what I want for you or for anyone.

I believe passionately in our need for pleasure of all kinds, including the enjoyment we get from food. I want you to eat nourishing food not because of its nutrient content but because it's so delicious. I want you to take time to enjoy your food and savor each bite. I want eating to be something you look forward to, not because you need it to fulfill an unmet emotional need but because you're hungry and the healthful meal you're getting ready to eat looks and tastes amazing. I want eating to be even more pleasurable for you than it has been, and without the extra serving of guilt, shame, and regret.

While tapping is often the fastest and most effective way to re-create your relationship with food and your body, I also want to share some tips clients have found useful for making eating a pleasure-infused experience.

**1. Before you begin eating, take three deep breaths and notice how you feel.** If you feel guilt, anger, frustration, or any other negative emotion, do some tapping before you begin eating. Then choose the emotions you're putting on your plate. I no longer eat ice cream and guilt. All of the food I eat, including ice cream, comes with a side of love and gratitude.

**2. Eat slowly and chew consciously.** So many of us are living fast-paced, action-packed lives. We're always searching for more time, so it's no wonder that we've developed a habit of inhaling our food, often chewing just enough—but no more—than we need to swallow it without choking. Taking time to eat more slowly gives you a chance to be aware of how you really feel. Being conscious about chewing your food has a big impact on how much pleasure you experience from your food. Also, because digestion begins in the mouth, when you chew your food thoroughly, your digestion also improves.

**3. Sit down while you eat.** Kitchen counters are meant for preparing food, not enjoying it. Kitchen sinks are meant for washing dishes, not for catching crumbs. When we eat while standing, we tend to feel rushed. Many of my biggest binges happened while I stood in front of my kitchen cabinet, holding the doors wide open. It would start with some nuts, then a cereal bar, maybe a few more nuts—but wait, I forgot about those pretzels. Okay, now I might as well open that bag of cookies and have one (or two) final handfuls of nuts. Inevitably, what started as a healthy snack turned into a binge. It's much easier to connect with how we feel, how hungry we really are, and how delicious our food tastes when we sit down at the table to enjoy the experience.

**4. Add other kinds of pleasure that relax and soothe you.** Pleasant and relaxing music, candlelight, nice cutlery, and pretty plates—all of these things add to the pleasure of your meal when guests come over. Why not do some of that for yourself? If you're short on time, just pick one additional source of pleasure that's fast and easy, like lighting a candle or putting on your favorite classical music. If it's music you're adding to your meal, just make sure it's calm and relaxing music, as fast and/or jarring music can act as a distraction, causing you to pay less attention to what you're eating and how it tastes.

**5. Be present and enjoy your food *without* distractions. (No TV, phone, or reading.)** When we're distracted by TV, reading a book or magazine, talking on the phone, or surfing the Internet, we can't fully enjoy and appreciate the food we're eating. Our brains numb out, quickly going on autopilot and preventing us from being conscious about what we're eating, how much we're eating, whether we're full, and—most important—how delicious our food tastes! It's time to be present with food and really enjoy it to the fullest.

As you read through these tips, did you notice any resistance? If these five simple guidelines feel impossible, ask yourself why and record your answers on a piece of paper or somewhere else you can refer back to. Your answers are tapping targets.

If you have young children, these guidelines may be more challenging. If that's the case, focus on working toward them and bringing as much presence to your eating as you can.

For others, these tips may seem overly simplistic and easy to just skim over, but being fully present with myself and my food as I'm eating has been one of the biggest game changers in my own weight loss and body confidence journey.

When we begin to practice this new way of being with food, we realize that we've avoided being present with food. This is because when we choose to be present, we also become present to our negative self-talk and emotions. It's important that we allow ourselves to be present with these uncomfortable voices and emotions and then do tapping to clear them instead of turning to food for comfort.

Just by following these simple guidelines, Jill realized that eating without the TV made her feel lonely. Then her negative self-talk about being single would come up. When she used tapping to address the belief that eating alone meant she was a "loser," she was able to release her judgment and enjoy her own company. She explained that she felt a shift by simply tapping as a surge of emotions came up.

Michelle realized that she felt guilty every time she took time for herself. She believed she needed to be productive while she ate, whether that meant reading a book or answering e-mails on her phone. When she felt this guilt, she wrote down all the thoughts that ran through her mind when she took time with her food. Then she simply read the list out loud while she tapped.

In the next chapter, we'll dive a little deeper in our efforts to figure out what got us to this point. We'll look at the events that occurred in our past, so we can understand better how they have affected us. But first, let's do a tapping meditation around being present with food and making eating a more pleasurable experience.

# Overcoming Emotional Eating

**Karate Chop:** Even though I don't feel like I have control over what I eat, I love and accept myself. (*Repeat three times.*)

**Eyebrow:** All this stress around food . . .

**Side of Eye:** I want to eat better . . .

**Under Eye:** But I don't want to deprive myself.

**Under Nose:** I need this food.

**Chin:** I have to keep eating when I'm not hungry . . .

**Collarbone:** Because I need a break.

**Under Arm:** I need an escape.

**Top of Head:** I need this food.

**Eyebrow:** Food has been such a comfort.

**Side of Eye:** Food is always there for me.

**Under Eye:** I'm not willing to let go of these unhealthy habits.

**Under Nose:** These intense cravings . . .

**Chin:** This inner battle around what to eat . . .

**Collarbone:** I don't want to eat in a destructive way.

**Under Arm:** But I don't want to deprive myself, either.

**Top of Head:** Maybe there's another way.

**Eyebrow:** Maybe I can still enjoy food.

**Side of Eye:** Maybe I can feel calm before I reach for food.

**Under Eye:** Maybe there are other ways to reward myself.

**Under Nose:** Maybe this is easier than I thought.

**Chin:** I'm open to finding new ways to reward myself.

**Collarbone:** I'm open to new ways to find comfort.

**Under Arm:** I choose to feel calm and centered now.

**Top of Head:** I find healthy ways to nurture myself.

**Eyebrow:** I am in tune with my body.

**Side of Eye:** It's been under so much stress.

**Under Eye:** This overeating is only draining my body.

**Under Nose:** I find ways to recharge through loving thoughts.

**Chin:** I'm kind to my body.

**Collarbone:** I choose foods that nourish my body.

**Under Arm:** I find the pleasure in healthy foods.

**Top of Head:** They feel good to my body and soul.

**Eyebrow:** I am in tune with what my body needs.

**Side of Eye:** I hydrate my body with pure, cleansing water.

**Under Eye:** I take deep breaths before I begin to eat.

**Under Nose:** I am present and in control.

**Chin:** I enjoy my food.

**Collarbone:** I am in control.

**Under Arm:** I know when I am full.

**Top of Head:** I make eating even more pleasurable . . .

**Eyebrow:** By being present and calm when I eat.

**Side of Eye:** This is easier than I thought.

**Under Eye:** I can be easy on myself.

**Under Nose:** I begin to incorporate healthy habits every day.

**Chin:** This feels so good.

**Collarbone:** I find the pleasure in healthy choices.

**Under Arm:** I am in control.

**Top of Head:** I nurture my body today with positive thoughts and nourishing foods.

# Chapter 5

# How Events Impact Weight and Body Confidence

On and off over the past 35 years, Holly had turned to bingeing in times of extreme stress. Although she had sought various forms of help with weight loss and had success, she had never been able to keep the weight off for more than a few years at a time. More than three decades later, she found herself losing hope that she could one day lose the weight for good.

About a month into my online weight loss class, Holly had a major breakthrough. While tapping, she realized that her bingeing had begun when she was eight years old. That was when her mother returned to work full time, and soon afterward, her dad had left. Afraid of living alone with her mother, a strict and unforgiving disciplinarian, Holly was angry at being abandoned by the one parent capable of expressing love and affection. Feeling like she had nowhere to turn, she began overeating, finding short-lived but much-needed comfort in bingeing.

Like Holly, most of us don't recognize the impact events have had on us until years, even decades, later, when we begin unraveling the areas of our lives where we feel dissatisfied. Through tapping, we

> No one feels strong when she examines her own weakness. But in facing weakness, you learn how much there is in you, and you find a blueprint for real strength.
>
> —PAT SUMMITT

can break down internal barriers and clear the damaging residue of the events that continue to affect us and our relationship with our weight and body. Holly started by giving her eight-year-old self an opportunity to say out loud how she really felt as she tapped. With tears streaming down her face, she felt an incredible release, and she was amazed that afterward she could recall the same memory without feeling overwhelmed by sadness. She felt a newfound compassion for herself and the little girl who simply sought much-needed comfort in food. This led to a new relationship with herself and with food. Having become more aware of her own stress, she now uses tapping to relieve it and no longer feels controlled by the urge to overindulge in food that doesn't nourish her or make her feel good.

To see how events may have impacted your relationship with yourself and your weight, in this chapter we'll be exploring three possible triggering events: events that lead to weight gain, that distort the weight loss experience, and that you can't pinpoint. All of these can have major effects on your ability to lose weight.

## Events That Lead to Weight Gain

It was through daily tapping on what was happening when she first began gaining weight that Beverly lost her first 30 pounds. Without focusing on weight loss or ever feeling deprived, she saw the pounds just seem to fall off. For her, the weight gain had begun during what she once called "stepfamily hell," a ten-year span of time that started soon after marrying her husband, who was then living with his two teenage children from a prior marriage.

The challenges Beverly faced during that time seemed endless. While her teenage stepson sold drugs from their front porch, Beverly struggled to find a positive, nurturing place in her stepchildren's troubled lives. Her husband retreated further into denial about what was happening in their house, and she felt alone and unsupported, unsure how to have a healthy marriage under the circumstances. Also afraid that she was failing as a stepmother, she abandoned her dream of having her own children and went to great lengths to hide her pain from friends and family. Her only source of comfort during that time was food; and year after year, the pounds continued to pile on.

When Beverly used tapping to clear the emotional charge of her memories, her body and her eating effortlessly began to transform. Because she had cleared the negative emotional residue from those memories, the name "stepfamily hell" no longer felt right. It had been a challenging time, but she had also learned many important lessons from it.

Listening to Beverly's story, I was struck by how she had named her memories of that time. Although being specific tends to be the best approach with tapping, fortunately it's not always necessary to dissect each layer of a memory one by one. Instead, we can do tapping on how those memories make us feel by giving them a title and in so doing, clear the emotional charge behind them.

By naming memories in a way that sums up how the experience felt, as Beverly did when she chose the name "stepfamily hell," you can often clear the emotional charge behind a collection of connected memories more quickly. It was because Beverly had cleared the negative emotional charge from her memories that she was able to rename that period of time "the decade of the steps" instead. The key to her success was that she could recall that time in her life and not feel physical stress in the present moment.

THE POWER OF EVENTS BIG AND (SEEMINGLY) SMALL

Clients and students are often surprised to discover how deeply they have been affected by seemingly minor events in their lives. That was true for Victoria, who realized while tapping that six short words said to her nearly 30 years ago had sparked her own struggle with weight.

"You don't deserve to live here," her first post-college landlord had said to her nearly three decades ago. It was at that moment when Victoria began turning toward food for comfort, afraid that she was unworthy of the good things in her life as her landlord had suggested.

Remembering his words while she tapped, tears flowed down her cheeks. She sobbed through the sadness and anger she had long been holding inside.

Once she had tapped through those emotions, she could recall his insult without feeling upset. "I feel like a switch has flipped in my brain," she shared. If there is an event that resulted in the belief that you don't deserve good things in your life, you will sabotage yourself every time you feel something good beginning to happen. By tapping on the moment, Victoria found that she no longer resisted her own progress. Practically overnight she found herself looking forward to exercising each day, and she began making herself healthy meals that tasted great and made her body feel good. Losing weight had suddenly become so much easier and more enjoyable because she now felt that she deserved good things in her life.

I use memories, but I do not allow memories to use me.

—LORD SHIVA

The events that spark or reignite our struggle with weight often span a wide range. Some clients can link the start of their weight struggle to a major event such as the loss of a job, relationship troubles, or a diagnosis. Other clients, like Victoria, can pinpoint a specific moment in time when they began turning to food for comfort. Whether it's a hurtful comment, an unwanted sexual advance, or some other long-ago experience, we sometimes find that what once seemed like a small and fleeting moment has impacted us on a very deep level.

Tapping on these events can help you move past the emotions and beliefs they have instilled in you. There are a number of different techniques that can be used to tap on such an event: Direct tapping, Tell the Story tapping, and Movie tapping. You can try all of these and see which works best for you.

**Direct Tapping Technique:** When you want to tap directly on a past event, simply give the event a title that helps you access the feelings you had at the time: "getting that look," "the hellish divorce," "losing the job," and so on.

When you think about this event, what is your strongest emotion? You may have a variety of emotions, which is fine, but for now focus on the one that grabs most of your attention.

When you think of the event, how intense is that emotion on a scale of 0 to 10? Begin tapping by filling in the blanks with the title and emotion.

Even though _____ made me feel _____, I love and accept myself.

Even though _____ made me feel _____, I love and accept myself.

Even though _____ made me feel _____, I love and accept myself.

*Continue tapping while saying the title, what happened, and how it made you feel until you can think of the event without experiencing emotional intensity. Be patient with yourself, as events often have multiple layers you may need to tap on.*

**Tell the Story Technique:** If you call your friend to complain about something that happened to you, you are telling the story. For this technique, pretend you're sharing a story with a friend and talk about what happened while you tap through the points.

*Bonus:* Once you feel calm and can tell the story without feeling an emotional charge, ask yourself, *If there was a positive lesson from this experience, what would it be?*

**Movie Technique:** The Movie Technique was developed by Gary Craig, the founder of EFT, as a way to address specific events rather than global issues. To do it, you run a movie of what took place in your mind. Creating a movie of an event pretty much guarantees that you are dealing with just one specific event. A movie has a beginning and an end. There are central characters who do and say specific things, and there is a usually a "crescendo" or peak moment in the movie.

The following questions will help you to set the stage for your short movie:

- *Could you make a short movie of this event?* One great thing about this technique is that at no point in this movie is it necessary for you to tell or say the details out loud. The critical part is the effects those details and any people involved have on the five senses. Focus on the sights, sounds, emotions, and physical feelings the characters are experiencing and what they are thinking and even smelling or tasting. One thing I do with clients when a movie feels too intense is have them imagine it in black and white and picture themselves sitting in the back row of the movie theater. Once they feel more comfortable with the black-and-white movie, they can add in color and lessen the distance between themselves and the movie screen.

- *How long would the movie last?* You want to make sure it is a short movie, three minutes or less. Often the key traumatic event in the movie is only seconds long. If there are several traumatic moments in the movie, break the movie down into as many small pieces as necessary to address each specific upsetting event.

- *What would the title be?* Create a name that is specific to that movie segment.

Now let's turn your specific event into a short movie with a title:

- Run the movie in your mind and evaluate the intensity you are having *now* (as you imagine it) on a scale of 0 to 10. You can also *guess* what your intensity would be if you vividly imagined it.

- Next, do several rounds of tapping on *"this _____ movie."* Check back on the intensity; typically it will have come down by several points.

- Now run the movie in your mind again, starting from a point that has no intensity or very low intensity, and make sure to *stop whenever you feel any intensity*. This is very important! Most of us have lived with traumas from the past for so long that we don't even notice that we push ourselves through the story regardless of how we feel. Not anymore! With EFT, when we recognize these moments of intensity, we can use them as opportunities for tapping.

- Run through the movie in your mind again, beginning to end, stopping to tap on any intense aspects as they come up. Keep tapping until you can play the entire movie without any change in it.

- Finally, run the movie again, this time exaggerating the sights, sounds, and colors. Really try to get upset about it. If you find some intensity coming back up, stop and tap again!

*Note:* It can be helpful to describe the movie out loud. Be sure to stop at any point that is upsetting—even just a little bit—and tap again until you are at 0. Then continue your movie narration.

As we explore more deeply how past events may be shaping your relationship with your weight, let's look next at the flip side of your weight loss journey—what may have happened as a result of prior weight loss.

## Events That Distort the Weight Loss Experience

Abby was in the best shape of her life, exercising often and eating healthfully. When she received a cancer diagnosis, it was the last thing she expected. Overwhelmed by the shock of her illness, she abandoned her healthy lifestyle, and the pounds soon began to pile on. Although years have passed since the traumatic diagnosis and her logical mind knows that her healthy lifestyle didn't lead to cancer, she finds herself resisting weight loss and healthy habits, afraid on some level that those habits will backfire as they seemed to last time.

So often, the lasting emotional impacts events have on us don't mesh with what our logical minds know to be true—that weight loss and healthy habits work for us, not against us. What happens is that we attribute meanings to events that happen simultaneously, like Abby's cancer diagnosis and her healthy lifestyle. That was also the case for Suzie, whose relationship with her weight was thrown off by a girl-friend's negative feedback. The last time she lost the weight, her friend accused her of thinking she was better than everyone else. Feeling alone and unsupported, Suzie quickly began regaining the weight, figuring that it was better to fit in by being overweight than to be thin and alone.

Take a moment now to ask yourself, *What happened the last time I lost weight and/or felt healthy?* Feel free to write down what you discover and then use it as your tapping target.

If nothing comes to mind, there's no need to worry. Simply continue reading.

If an event does come to mind, you can tap on it using the techniques we just learned. This tapping script may help you get started. Rate the emotional intensity of the event before you begin tapping.

**Karate Chop:** Even though something bad happened the last time I lost weight, I love and accept myself and I am safe. (*Repeat three times.*)

**Eyebrow:** This bad thing that happened . . .

**Side of Eye:** I was feeling so good . . .

**Under Eye:** And it backfired.

**Under Nose:** This resistance to losing weight again . . .

**Chin:** Part of me wants to . . .

**Collarbone:** Part of me doesn't.

**Under Arm:** I don't want to repeat what happened.

**Top of Head:** It doesn't feel safe to lose weight.

*When the intensity of your initial tapping target is 5 or lower, you can move on to the positive.*

**Eyebrow:** Maybe this time can be different . . .

**Side of Eye:** Maybe it was never about the weight . . .

**Under Eye:** It's always been about me.

**Under Nose:** I have learned so much from the past experience.

**Chin:** I take the lessons . . .

**Collarbone:** And release the pain.

**Under Arm:** This time will be different.

**Top of Head:** I feel safe and confident within my power.

*Take a deep breath and check in with how you feel. Measure the intensity again and continue tapping until you experience relief.*

## Events You Can't Pinpoint

Sometimes weight slowly becomes a problem as the stress in our lives builds. When that's the case, there is no need to remember a specific event or period of time to get results. These questions are just a way to start getting clear on what may be holding you back. If you don't have a specific event, you can still experience a major shift by tapping on beliefs, which we'll begin doing in the next chapter.

Even if you're not sure if this chapter is relevant to you, I recommend that you finish it and do the tapping exercises as well. Through tapping you may discover memories that were buried and clear them quickly, lowering the stress that can interfere with weight loss.

# When Words Hurt

"You're fat, and no one is going to listen to you if you're fat." That was the advice my former mentor gave me when I was 20 years old, volunteering at the wellness and nutrition conference he was facilitating.

As the two young men standing nearby looked down in embarrassment, I quickly blurted out, "My weight isn't stopping me—I still get guys."

While that wasn't quite accurate, it was all I could think to say after being attacked so unexpectedly. "That's because you have big boobs," my mentor replied.

Speechless and desperate for a way out, I was shocked when he continued. "I'm just saying this because if you want to make an impact in this world and speak on stage, being fat will take away from your message. People will only be able to focus on your weight."

Looking back on that moment, I understand that his words hurt me as deeply as they did because I believed them even before he said them. Instead of having the appropriate response of healthy anger and not tolerating such an obscenely unnecessary attack, I let those words tear me down because I felt they were true. I had already spent years obsessing over my body, making it into *the* obstacle standing between me and my future.

Because I felt powerless to change my weight or even express my anger, I quickly resorted to rebellion. I told myself that I would prove him wrong and become successful without losing weight. If I lost weight, I would be proving him right—and that was unacceptable. So instead of processing my feelings in a healthy way, I buried them once again with food. This time, I told myself, not losing weight felt right, like I was standing up for women who feel judged for not fitting into a size 2 dress. In fact, by trying to eat my feelings away, I was only hurting myself more.

Looking back now, I see how wrong my former mentor was; there are incredible women who change the world without fitting into a size

2. And even as I tried to prove him wrong, I was still allowing his words to impact me. The key was to let go of what he had said so I could act in a way that was best for *me*. Finding the best ways to rebel against him—or make him happy, for that matter—could never serve me. The journey to true body confidence needs to be about meeting our own needs and desires, not about accepting or rejecting other people's ideas.

When we use tapping to clear the emotional impact of hurtful words that have been hurled at us, we sometimes need to first process multiple levels of the same experience. One student in my class announced one day several weeks into the program that she had made a major breakthrough. After being told by her late husband that no one would ever love her because she was too fat, she shared that she finally loved herself at a deeper level and was ready for romantic love. Then she added that she was ready to "prove him wrong."

> The knowledge of the past stays with us. To let go is to release the images and emotions, the grudges and fears, the clingings and disappointments of the past that bind our spirit.
>
> —JACK KORNFIELD

I quickly pointed out that if she had the belief she needed to prove him wrong, she would never take care of herself and lose the weight she so badly wanted to lose. She would unconsciously rebel against losing weight because losing weight would mean her husband was right: that men could only value her for her body. If her weight loss journey was about him or men in general, not about her, long-term weight loss would feel like an uphill battle. I suggested that, using tapping, she continue to process and clear the emotional scars her late husband's hurtful words had left. Once she felt committed to weight loss purely for herself, she would be able to embark on a pleasurable and rewarding weight loss journey.

## RELEASING THE PAIN OF HURTFUL WORDS PEOPLE SAY

I felt so wounded and ashamed by what my former mentor said that years passed before I could share the story with anyone. Just remembering the words—"You're fat, and no one is going to listen to what you have to say"—created a lump in my throat as my eyes welled with tears. The memory was too painful to face, so I did everything I could to avoid it, even though the pain of that moment felt so real and ever present.

We've already discussed how to tap through the emotions of painful words in regard to emotional eating in the moment. But tapping on these hurtful events is possible even long after they have taken place. As painful as memories of hurtful words may be, when we react to recalling these memories with big emotional surges, we're perfectly positioned to use tapping to clear the pain.

> Our parents, our children, our spouses, and our friends will continue to press every button we have, until we realize what it is that we don't want to know about ourselves, yet. They will point us to our freedom every time.
>
> —BYRON KATIE

When painful memories send you back in time, the amygdala in your brain goes on high alert, preparing to protect you from danger. What you need to do is train the amygdala so it recognizes that these memories are not actually dangerous. By tapping on the hurtful words that someone said to you, you're giving your brain new instructions, telling it that the memory is no longer threatening—that you can now feel safe when remembering those words.

Often when you clear a significant emotional burden, you will experience a physical release, such as crying or shaking. As you continue tapping through your memory, you will find that the hurtful words lose their power. For me, once a stream of tears had rolled down my cheeks, I could say the words he had said to me and feel centered and relaxed. That was only possible because I had used tapping to release the emotional power of those words.

Let's do some tapping on the hurtful words people have said to you. Begin tapping while repeating the words until you can say them and feel calm in the moment. Feel free to fill in the blanks below to create a personalized tapping script. If it's easier to begin by writing them down on a separate piece of paper, you're welcome to do that.

**Karate Chop:** Even though _____ said _____, I love and accept myself. (*Repeat three times.*)

**Eyebrow:** _____

**Side of Eye:** _____

**Under Eye:** _____

**Under Nose:** _____

**Chin:** _____

**Collarbone:** _____

**Under Arm:** _____

**Top of Head:** _____

*We are often too quick to jump to forcing ourselves to forgive because we don't want to admit how much the words hurt. It's okay to be angry; express that anger as you tap. Don't move to the positive unless the positive statements feel true.*

**Eyebrow:** Those words don't have power over me . . .

**Side of Eye:** Unless I give them power.

**Under Eye:** I take my power back.

**Under Nose:** If they are this hard on me . . .

**Chin:** I can only imagine how hard they are on themselves.

**Collarbone:** Their words are not a reflection of me . . .

**Under Arm:** Their words are a reflection of themselves.

**Top of Head:** I have compassion for what they must be going through.


## MOVING TOWARD COMPASSION

As we clear the emotional sting of hurtful words through tapping, it's helpful to guide ourselves toward a place of compassion for the person or people who have hurt us. This is difficult, if not impossible, if you haven't yet cleared the full emotional charge of their hurtful words. If you experience any resistance to this idea, that's an indication that you need to keep tapping on the words.

I often end tapping sessions that are focused on clearing emotions created by hurtful words with "If they are this hard on me, I can only imagine how hard they must be on themselves." When I did this process with a client whose mother had always wanted her to be a Southern belle, she cringed at how harsh her mother's own self-talk must be.

Feeling compassion for the person who said hurtful words to you makes forgiveness a gentle process and allows you to take your power back in a warm and loving way.

I'd like to stress again, though, that too often we try to jump too quickly into compassion. Allow yourself to feel angry or hurt while you tap. Only when you feel like you can say those words without a physical reaction can you begin to open up to compassion and forgiveness.


## PROCESSING DAILY EVENTS

Small events we experience every day often take a toll on our health and well-being, so it's best to nip these things in the bud as they're happening rather than letting them build up over the years. So as you go through your day, try to notice events and comments that create an emotional response. Whenever you experience negative emotions such as anxiety, anger, or hurt, take some time to tap on them.

For example, you could experience something like this: after you've been working long hours for weeks, your boss sends you a harsh e-mail and you're furious. You get home angry and all you want to do is shut out the world by grabbing a snack and getting comfortable on the couch. Instead of snapping at your family and inhaling your food, you can use tapping to process your emotional response to your boss's e-mail. It can often be as simple as reading the e-mail to yourself while you tap. This will help clear the event before it can have a large negative impact on you.

The next step in your process of looking within focuses on limiting beliefs, which can restrict what you think is possible in your life. But before you dive into beliefs, I suggest you first do a tapping meditation on how events may have impacted your journey up to this point.

# Setting Yourself Free from the Past

**Karate Chop:** Even though I've allowed these events to hold me back, I love and accept myself and set myself free. (*Repeat three times.*)

**Eyebrow:** Looking closer can feel overwhelming . . .

**Side of Eye:** It's easier to ignore my past . . .

**Under Eye:** It's easier to ignore these events . . .

**Under Nose:** But they are impacting me daily.

**Chin:** Life doesn't feel so easy . . .

**Collarbone:** With these past events weighing on me.

**Under Arm:** Maybe I can look closer . . .

**Top of Head:** By being gentle and curious.

**Eyebrow:** These events that happened to me . . .

**Side of Eye:** I've used them as proof . . .

**Under Eye:** To hold myself back.

**Under Nose:** Those words they said . . .

**Chin:** I've allowed myself to believe them.

**Collarbone:** All these past events . . .

**Under Arm:** I allow myself to become aware of them . . .

**Top of Head:** And give a voice to how I feel.

**Eyebrow:** The story I've been telling myself . . .

**Side of Eye:** As to why I can't succeed . . .

**Under Eye:** I've used these events as evidence . . .

**Under Nose:** That I can't do it . . .

**Chin:** That I'm not enough.

**Collarbone:** Maybe I'm more than these events . . .

**Under Arm:** Taking my power back from the past . . .

**Top of Head:** Feeling my power in the moment.

**Eyebrow:** These hurtful words from the past . . .

**Side of Eye:** I've allowed them to live on in my mind.

**Under Eye:** What they said was a reflection on them.

**Under Nose:** I release the power these words had on me . . .

**Chin:** And begin to listen to my own words . . .

**Collarbone:** That tell me all the reasons why I am enough.

**Under Arm:** I listen to my own voice . . .

**Top of Head:** That guides me forward.

**Eyebrow:** These past events . . .

**Side of Eye:** I take the lessons . . .

**Under Eye:** And release any pain.

**Under Nose:** I'm grateful for all I've learned . . .

**Chin:** Maybe I was rejected . . .

**Collarbone:** So I could be redirected to something better.

**Under Arm:** I am open to discovering . . .

**Top of Head:** All the hidden blessings in these past events.

**Eyebrow:** All those moments have led me to this moment . . .

**Side of Eye:** When I choose love . . .

**Under Eye:** When I choose joy . . .

**Under Nose:** When I see my own worth.

**Chin:** I am so grateful for my past.

**Collarbone:** I am grateful for all I've learned.

**Under Arm:** I take all these empowering lessons from my past . . .

**Top of Head:** And set myself free.

# Chapter 6

# The Power of Beliefs

In her book *You Can Heal Your Life* (which has sold more than 50 million copies!), Louise Hay shares one of her key philosophies: "The only thing we are ever dealing with is a thought, and a thought can be changed." As we begin looking at how beliefs impact the weight loss journey, we must start by understanding that a belief is a thought we have over and over again.

In this chapter we'll see how much beliefs impact experience and can limit us (or support us) in the journey toward body confidence and weight loss. When a client tells me she hates herself and her body, for instance, she is actually saying that she hates her belief about herself, which might be "I'm not good enough." *This thought, this belief about herself, produces an emotion. That emotion then creates a stress response in her body that makes her belief seem valid.*

With tapping, you can change your beliefs by targeting the emotions and the stress response your beliefs create by focusing on the belief itself. Once that stress response is lowered or gone altogether, the old negative belief—"I'm not good enough"—no longer feels true. You can then create a positive belief that does feel true, helps you love yourself, and creates positive momentum for you on your weight loss and body confidence journey.

# How Beliefs Affect Your Experience

Before we discuss beliefs in greater detail, let's look at the relationship between beliefs and experiences. Louise Hay again sums it up perfectly in *You Can Heal Your Life:* "No matter what the problem is, our experiences are just outer effects of inner thoughts." In other words, experiences are reflections of beliefs. To put it another way, your beliefs are your blueprint for the world.

If you have a negative belief like "I'm not good enough," you can't feel happy or experience real pleasure. Believing that you're not good enough (or that you're not beautiful/smart/strong enough) is like giving yourself a life sentence; it leaves no room for any other possibility. With that belief in mind, you unconsciously look for evidence to support that belief and take action (or refrain from action) that supports it. You interpret events in ways that support the belief even when it causes you pain. You also unconsciously seek out or are attracted to people who give you the kind of negative feedback that "proves" your belief.

The idea that beliefs create experience hit home for me one day several years ago when I shared with my friend Brenna what some guy had randomly said to me: "You'd be cute if you lost some weight." It was yet another cruel and unsolicited comment about my weight, and again I was devastated. Knowing my history of being a target for comments like this, she looked right at me and said, "This is not normal, Jess. People don't say mean things like that to most people." As I thought about what she had said, I realized that I had been holding on to a belief in my body that *I* wasn't good enough. For years I'd been unconsciously attracting and seeking out people who confirmed that belief. I also found myself rejecting and playing down compliments and only focusing on the times people told me I wasn't good enough.

If you believe you aren't worthy in your current body, you will gravitate toward people who reflect that belief back to you. When you don't believe those things about yourself, you no longer tolerate people who treat you in a disrespectful way. Instead, because you believe you deserve love and support, you're able to love and support yourself first and then cultivate a supportive community of people who can also love and support you.

When I began tapping on my belief that I wasn't good enough in my current body, I was able to clear the emotions and stress response this belief had created in me. It didn't happen overnight. I had to break down all the different events I was using as proof that the belief was true. (You can see in this example what we saw earlier in the Tapping Tree—that symptoms, emotions, events, and beliefs are often interconnected.)

What began happening in the weeks and months that followed was amazing. I started to gravitate away from people who were judgmental and negative and toward relationships that supported the new positive beliefs I had created about myself. My entire life soon began to transform, and the weight began falling off faster than it ever had. And it all happened without focusing on weight loss or feeling deprived. Because I had created a new belief that allowed me to love myself, I was naturally making better decisions and no longer needed dieting and extreme exercise to lose weight and punish my body. Instead, I could trust myself and my body and still lose weight—and that is exactly what happened.

I see this same pattern repeat itself again and again in my clients. They're amazed by how easy weight loss feels once they've used tapping to change their beliefs about themselves, their bodies, and their weight loss journeys.

## The Key to Identifying Your Beliefs—Question Everything!

Holding on to negative beliefs is like wearing dark-tinted glasses all day, every day. When we're wearing them, everything in our world seems scary and threatening. But when we take them off and put on clear glasses—which, in this case, means creating positive beliefs—the world around us seems brighter. Suddenly we feel hopeful, able to naturally seek out experiences that make us feel good.

As much pain as negative beliefs can cause, we aren't always taught to evaluate them. Whether we adopted them from our immediate environment or they were passed down to us from our parents, they often appear disguised as facts. We may question authority and examine beliefs during our teenage years, but as we get older we tend to settle into beliefs and think what we believe is just how the world is—and, more dangerously, *This is just who I am.*

> The important thing is not to stop questioning. Curiosity has its own reason for existence.
>
> —ALBERT EINSTEIN

Targeting a belief begins with first questioning the way we have been viewing the world and ourselves. When we tap while focusing on the belief, its emotional stronghold weakens and we have the ability to take a step back and ask ourselves, *Is this really true?* Then we have the freedom to choose a more empowering belief that supports us in creating the life (and weight loss journey) we want to have.

At first, we may resist and distrust the idea that by changing our beliefs we can change our lives. After all, we think, we have so much evidence to prove that what we believe is true. For starters, we've never been able to lose weight without depriving ourselves, counting calories, dieting, and subjecting ourselves to extreme exercise that feels like punishment. That is the truth; that is what happened, so why pretend otherwise?

While this seems logical and may initially feel true, that resistance we feel is most often rooted in the stress response that a negative belief has created in us. Until we do tapping to clear that stress response, we can't create a new experience for ourselves. If we shut out the possibility that weight loss can be pleasurable, for example, we are closing ourselves off to having a positive weight loss experience.

Often when clients come to understand that their beliefs are just thoughts that they can change, they realize that their disempowering beliefs don't even seem logically true. They'll often say, "I know that belief isn't true. I don't even want to believe it but it just *feels* so true." We saw that in the last chapter with Abby, whose cancer diagnosis created a disempowering belief that losing weight and being healthy had led to her illness. She knew that wasn't the case but couldn't seem to get rid of the *feeling* that it was. When she used tapping to clear the emotions and stress response that had been validating her belief, she could let go of it. That same principle applies to everyone: until we clear the emotion and stress response behind negative beliefs, we can't fully let go of them.

The first step in releasing negative beliefs is to identify them, and we do that by learning to question everything, including what we've always known as "facts." That's what we'll do next.

So take a moment to ask yourself the following questions. You may want to write them down, along with your answers.

- What negative feedback have I been replaying from others to support my limiting beliefs?

- When did I learn that I'm not (good/pretty/smart) enough?

- What events have I used as proof to support my negative beliefs?

## Getting Clear on Your Story

As we begin to identify limiting beliefs, we often find that we have many of them and that they are spread across different areas of our lives. Over time these beliefs become the larger story we're telling ourselves about who we are and what's possible for us. Once we use tapping to address the limiting beliefs that have shaped our story, we can create a new story and make incredible progress in ways that feel natural and enjoyable.

That's what happened when Lori discovered her own story and used tapping to clear her negative beliefs. "I went from obsessing about weight loss to obsessing about self-love. I realized that self-love was the key. I kept finding ways to take care of myself. Suddenly exercise and eating well became fulfilling and exciting. When I changed my beliefs about what it took to lose weight—and more important, what I believed about myself—losing weight and taking care of myself became easy and fun."

Just as you used the Tell the Story technique in the last chapter to clear events, you can use that same technique to clear limiting beliefs. Let's look at the story you may be telling yourself and then do some tapping to clear the way for new beliefs that support you and your weight loss journey.

DISCOVER YOUR STORY

The first part of this exercise involves writing, and then we begin tapping.

Start by finishing the two sentences below, which will help you see your own limiting beliefs. Write each sentence down and complete it in your own words.

- I can't lose weight/be thin because . . .
- I want to lose weight but . . . .

Write down the beliefs you discovered by finishing these sentences. These are your tapping targets.

When you pinpoint a belief, say it out loud and ask yourself, on a scale of 0 to 10, *How true does this feel?* If it feels like a simple fact, it would be a 10. Then begin tapping while telling your story. A helpful setup statement may be "Even though I believe (state your belief here), I accept myself and how I feel, and I am open to a new way of thinking."

We'll explore the limiting beliefs within your story throughout the rest of this chapter and then learn how to tap on them.

Clients often tell me that when they tap on the story they've been telling themselves, they start to see their lives in a whole new way. They realize that they've used various events to support their limiting beliefs. Once they use tapping to clear their old beliefs, they can see events in their past in a new light and even discover a valuable lesson or hidden blessing in them.

To explore your story in more depth, you also need to look at your beliefs about yourself, your genetics, your body, and your weight loss journey.

## Beliefs about Your Genetics

Growing up on an island off Scotland with a population of fewer than 100 people, Marjorie was an anomaly within her family. Since childhood she had been the only one among her seven siblings who was overweight. The consensus within the community was that she had inherited "bad genes" from her aunt, who had also always been overweight. "I felt like I had grabbed the shortest straw in the gene pool," she explained. Those "bad genes" became part of who Marjorie was, a fact that she didn't have the power to change.

Many of us who come from families where weight issues are common also point to genetics as the cause of our struggles with weight. "See," we say, "this is just who I am." At other times we may blame genetics because we're tired of blaming ourselves and we feel exhausted by our unsuccessful attempts at dieting. The idea that we are victims of our genetics is not only scientifically inaccurate; it also strips us of the power to change.

Blaming the body is like blaming a car that won't run when in fact we never bothered to give it the proper fuel and loving maintenance. The truth is that we don't need to blame anyone or anything for our weight issues; the key is to replace blame with curiosity. Several weeks into my class, Marjorie began to do that and had an exciting breakthrough. By tapping on her beliefs about her body, she realized that she had grown up in a culture and family where food was an expression of love. Her aunt loved to bake, and piling people's plates high with food expressed how much she cared for them. All these years later, Marjorie realized, she had been "eating" love in the form of baked cookies, scones, muffins, and cakes.

When we point to a family that is overweight, we don't need to look at genetics but instead at the food habits within that family. We can then ask ourselves what beliefs we may have unconsciously adopted around eating, food, and weight. When we stop blaming the body, we can change our emotions, stress levels, and behavior as well as how the body functions.

Genetics obviously play a role in the body, but if we believe that we have no control over gene expression, it's easy to give up and surrender to unhealthy habits that match the disappointment we feel. You have more power over gene expression than you think. Let's take a look at the science behind that claim.

## THE SCIENCE OF GENETICS

"We're going to miss our flight," I whispered to Nick Polizzi, director of *The Tapping Solution* movie and the longtime friend of my brother Nick.

"I know," he replied, "but this is *so* worth it." I nodded, excited to keep going with the interview.

We'd arrived at Bruce Lipton's house a couple of hours earlier, ready to conduct an hour-long interview with this highly acclaimed scientist who is also a top-selling author. We assumed he'd be stiff and formal—scientist-like—but from the start he was one great surprise after another. He greeted us with a big smile at the front door of his house in the San Jose hills in a T-shirt and shorts. As we started setting up our camera equipment, he turned to me and said, "Let me know when you're ready to start and I'll put on a nicer shirt." I was shocked by how casual and friendly he was—so different from the reserved scientist in a lab coat I had imagined.

I'd done extensive research in advance of the interview and knew how much Bruce's work has revolutionized our understanding of how beliefs impact the body. In 1967, decades before the rest of us knew what it was, Bruce was already doing stem-cell research. He had started in that field while earning his Ph.D. in developmental cell biology under the mentorship of Dr. Irwin R. Konigsberg, one of the first scientists ever to successfully clone stem cells.

The pioneering work Bruce has done in the decades since has shown us that genes don't predict health, success, happiness, or weight. In fact, gene expression is based on environment. That environment extends beyond particles and molecules to include emotions and beliefs. In other words, we can change how our cells develop and function by changing our beliefs, stress levels, and nutrition.

> Genetics loads the gun, but environment pulls the trigger!
>
> —DR. JUDITH STERN

By the time we left his house, two and a half hours had passed. Every moment we had spent with Bruce Lipton had been amazing. It was, and still is, my favorite interview from the movie. Talking to him was fascinating, and by the end Nick Polizzi and I felt like giant sponges soaked to maximum capacity with incredible new knowledge.

Since we'd already missed our flight home, Nick and I had no choice but to drive six hours to Los Angeles and catch a different one. During that drive, we talked at length about Bruce's work. It's really a pretty amazing idea—that our beliefs, emotions, stress, and nutrition can change how cells behave and function. His work shows us that we're not victims of genetics but instead products of our thoughts. According to this way of thinking, there are only very rare and occasional instances when genetics play a significant role in our ability to overcome weight struggles. While this puts a lot of power in our hands to change our own lives and, for example, create an easier and more enjoyable weight loss journey, it also robs many of us of the excuse that our weight struggles come from "bad genes."

Take a moment now to think about the internal environment you're creating for yourself and your cells. Is your body living in one that is loving and nurturing, or an environment of self-hatred and punishment? Feel free to write down your thoughts.

Remember: the point of this process is not to blame anyone or anything—including yourself—for your past weight struggles. The point now is to get curious about your beliefs and how your internal environment may be impacting your weight loss journey.

Keep those questions and your responses in mind as we begin exploring beliefs around weight loss next.

To watch a segment of my interview with Bruce Lipton, go to www.TheTappingSolution.com/chapter6.

## Beliefs Around Weight Loss

"I really want to lose weight, but it doesn't seem worth it," Polly confessed in our first coaching session. Losing weight and being thin, for Polly, had always been about deprivation and struggle. After weeks and months of dieting and hard work, the weight would come off, but even when she felt thin she couldn't enjoy herself. Always obsessing about calories and exercise, she worried about when the weight would return, which it inevitably did. As much as she still wanted to lose weight, she couldn't stand the thought of going through the process all over again. Absolutely nothing about the experience of losing weight had ever been enjoyable.

Polly's experience is incredibly common, and like most beliefs, the belief that weight loss is about struggle and deprivation quickly turns into reality. If you believe you must suffer to lose weight, you will either fail to lose it or you will drop a few pounds but regain them soon afterward. I'll say it again: our bodies can't be healthy and thrive when they're constantly being scrutinized and subjected to a stressful internal environment.

One of the most common responses I hear from women who follow my online weight loss program is "I'm losing weight and I don't feel deprived!" They're amazed, but why is deprivation-free weight loss such a shock? Since diets typically don't look at the underlying beliefs and emotions that lead us toward self-sabotaging behaviors, in many ways they set us up to fail. Relying on diet and exercise alone, we're forced to use willpower as our sole source of motivation, and that makes weight loss feel difficult.

If you have a belief that it's hard to lose weight, you will continue to make it hard. If you have a belief that losing weight can be pleasurable, you can more easily adopt new behaviors such as eating more nourishing meals and exercising regularly. Take a moment now to explore your beliefs about weight loss and do some tapping on it.


## YOUR BELIEFS ABOUT WEIGHT LOSS

To begin exploring your own beliefs around weight loss, ask yourself the following question: "What if having a healthy and strong body could be a fun and pleasurable experience?"

Does this idea make you scoff or roll your eyes? Does it make you feel anxious or angry or frustrated? Write down any emotional reactions you have, whether it's resistance, self-blame, curiosity, excitement, or some other emotion. You can use these emotions that come up as tapping targets, but you can also look to tap directly on your beliefs.

To discover what these beliefs are, ask yourself the following questions and write down your answers.

1. What beliefs do you have about your genes and body?

    a) It's my genetics.

    b) I have a slow metabolism.

    c) My body is working against me.

    d) Other(s): _____

2. What are your beliefs around what it takes to be healthy and strong?

> a) If it's not hard, I'm not doing it right.
>
> b) I have to deprive myself.
>
> c) I have to eat perfectly.
>
> d) I have to suffer to see results.
>
> e) I have to obsess over calories.
>
> f) I need to criticize myself to "get my act together" and be healthier.
>
> g) Other(s): _____

I'll teach you later how to tap on these beliefs. For now, I just want you to identify them.

## Beliefs about Others

To this day Lisa remembers how much it hurt when the skinny girls in high school turned their attention toward her. They always seemed to have so much fun taunting and teasing Lisa about her weight. It seemed like their favorite pastime.

As we tapped on her memories, Lisa was able to release the emotional pain she had been holding inside for all these years. During that process, she also realized that she had formed a belief in high school that all thin women are mean. Not wanting to become "one of them," she was shocked to realize all the ways she'd been unconsciously sabotaging her own weight loss for many years.

The judgments we make about others, especially other women, often seem like our dirty little secrets. Whether we voice them to a precious few friends or keep them to ourselves, our judgments feel bitter and shameful—but also completely true. It's not that we want to feel this way, we tell ourselves, it's that we can't help but form logical conclusions based on years of experience.

When we dig deeper, we see that our judgments are reflections of our own beliefs that contribute to self-sabotaging behaviors. I remember rolling my eyes years ago whenever I saw a physically fit woman running. I didn't understand why you would run unless you were being chased. I judged physically fit women as vain. The truth was that I was annoyed that I wasn't born with the "love to work out" gene. And if I couldn't be like them, at least I could judge them. Judging them somehow felt more empowering to me. I finally realized my judgments were a painful reflection of the limiting beliefs I had about myself and created a block to my own success.

Are there thin women who are vain and cruel and have a bad attitude and an unhealthy relationship with exercise? Of course there are. But there are also overweight women who are vain and cruel and have a bad attitude and an unhealthy relationship with exercise. There are 8 billion people on the planet. Weight and body mass index do not determine a person's attitude!

When you pass judgment on someone else, you are teaching your subconscious mind that it's not safe for you to have what they have because you may be judged in the same way you're judging them. So when you look at someone's Facebook picture and pass judgment on how easy life must be for them, you're telling yourself that it's not safe for your life to be easy or else you may be judged. Then you'll unconsciously continue to find ways to prove your value through struggling.

Instead of being judgmental when you see someone who has more money or a healthier body, get curious. Befriend them. Ask them what motivates them to stay healthy. More important, cheer them on. The more you can celebrate someone else's success, the more congruent you will be with creating similar success for yourself.

Take a moment now to think about how you judge others, including those little snap judgments you make while in line at the store, in meetings, with your neighbors, or when you see other parents at your child's school. Do you criticize other people more often than you praise and appreciate them? Do you tend to make big assumptions about who they are based on how they look or on little things they say or do?

## How Do You Judge Others?

To help you see how you may judge other women, here are some common beliefs my clients have discovered through this process. If any of these ring true, write them down and then write down any others that aren't listed below.

**The judgment:** She's so beautiful. She must be vain.

**What your subconscious hears:** I can never feel beautiful or people will think I'm vain. It's not safe to feel beautiful.

_____

**The judgment:** She might be thin but at least I'm nice.

**What your subconscious hears:** I either need to be thin or nice—I can't be both.

_____

**The judgment:** Skinny bitch!

**What your subconscious hears:** If I'm skinny I will be looked at as a bitch. It's not safe to be skinny.

_____

**The judgment:** Life must be so easy for her because she's thin.

**What your subconscious hears:** If I'm thin or if I make life easier, I will be seen as less valuable and I'll be judged. It's not safe to be thin. It's not safe to make life easy.

Once you've made an initial list of your judgments about others, you may find yourself discovering new and different judgments you make as you go about your day. There's no need to feel discouraged by this or to shame or blame yourself for being judgmental. The more aware you are of how you're seeing others, the more quickly you can uncover your own beliefs, do some tapping on them, and make positive changes in yourself and your life.

Now that we've explored how you may judge others, let's look at what you believe about yourself.

## Beliefs about Yourself

Every time Isabelle gained weight, she would get frustrated and say to herself, "God, I'm so stupid!" She'd continue by saying, "I know what I should be doing. I don't understand why I'm not doing it." I asked her one day why she was so quick to judge herself as stupid. As we did tapping on that, she remembered working in her father's office as a child, starting when she was only eight years old. He was a doctor, and every time she made a mistake, he would say, "What, are you stupid?" His words stayed with her into adulthood, and every time Isabelle made a mistake she called herself stupid. Over time, her failure to lose weight had become her biggest "mistake," a constant reminder of how stupid she must be.

As we did some tapping together to clear the emotions and stress behind her memory and the "You're stupid" belief it had created, Isabelle's mood lightened. Once we'd tapped through the emotional intensity of her belief, we continued tapping while asking each other, "What, are you stupid?" As soon as I asked her that, she replied, "No, but thanks for asking." Her old belief that she was stupid for not being able to lose weight had suddenly lost its power, and after several rounds of "What, are you stupid?" we both broke into laughter.

When we begin looking at how we judge ourselves, we're often shocked at the beliefs we've been carrying around. They're often things like *You're so stupid. You're a fat slob. You have no self-control. You never do*

> Nothing splendid has ever been achieved except by those who dared believe that something inside themselves was superior to circumstance.
>
> —BRUCE BARTON

*anything right. You can never stick to anything. You'll never be good enough.* As one client said to me, "My biggest Aha! moment was when I realized that if someone spoke to my five-year-old daughter the way I speak to myself, I would knock them out, so why am I speaking to myself like this?"

Our beliefs about ourselves sometimes leak out at random moments when we fall into old language patterns. One day I was filming a video with a friend. As she was struggling to set up a light, she muttered, "I'm so stupid." Without thinking, I yelled, "Hey! Don't talk about my friend like that!" We both looked at each other and burst out laughing as she pointed to me and said, "Good catch." We need to do our best to catch ourselves in these moments.

If you look at every time you eat a cookie or skip exercise as a mistake, you're reinforcing beliefs like *I never follow through with things, I can never lose weight,* and *Losing weight is impossible.* Such beliefs keep you locked inside your old self-destructive story. If you find yourself falling into an old self-sabotaging behavior but have the belief that you are smart, healthy, and worthy, you will quickly align yourself with your positive story about yourself and make a better and more empowering decision.

So what do you say to yourself when you make a mistake? If you respond with negative self-talk, you are more likely to make more bad decisions. Beating ourselves up for emotional eating doesn't stop the destructive pattern. If we believe these negative beliefs about ourselves, we will use that one binge to prove our point and continue to repeat the same habit because it seems congruent with who we think we are. If we have empowering beliefs about ourselves, we don't need to judge that experience of overeating. Instead, we can quickly move on to make a better decision.

The words *I am* are the two most powerful words in the human language. How we end that sentence determines our fate.

## Research: How Words Impact Performance

In a study done with college students, cognitive neuroscientist Sara Bengtsson discovered a link between expectations and performance. One group of students was given affirmative messages using words such as *smart*, *intelligent*, and *clever* before taking a test, while a second group was primed with negative words like *stupid* and *ignorant*. The group that was primed with positive words performed better on the test.

What's really interesting is how the better-performing group responded to making mistakes. When the group that was primed with positive words like *clever* was aware of having made a mistake, they showed increased activity in the anterior medial part of the prefrontal cortex, which is a region in the brain involved in self-reflection and recollection. The group that was primed with negative words like stupid showed no increase in brain activity when they made a mistake.

In other words, the belief that each group had about themselves had a huge impact on how they responded to making a mistake. Either the brain became activated to make a better decision next time or it showed no increased activity.

This same principle applies to your own self-talk. If you call yourself "fat" or "stupid," you're creating a negative expectation that your brain will make sure you fulfill. When you make a decision that isn't supporting your goal, you (and your brain) simply surrender to the limiting belief.

## Beliefs about Your Body

During our long struggle with our weight, many of us have come to see our own body as the enemy, something that needs to earn our love. Because it doesn't meet our strict and narrow cultural standard of beauty, it has become a source of constant misery, like a defect we can't seem to hide or fix. Its appearance is so awful to us that being happy inside our current body seems impossible. We have to lose the weight first, we tell ourselves, and then, once we're thin, we'll be able to feel good and enjoy ourselves.

The truth is that we have the process backward. As we've begun to see, to experience lasting weight loss—and just as important, to feel body confidence—we need to learn to love ourselves and our bodies first. Let's begin that process by discussing the negative beliefs you may have about your body.

While there are many different negative beliefs you may have about your body, I'm going to focus on the two most common ones I've seen in my clients and students:

- *There's nothing to appreciate about my body.*

- *I can't be happy and really live my life until I lose weight.*

Carly had lived with both of these body beliefs for as long as she could remember. Her weight loss attempts had been so frustrating that years ago she had undergone a very expensive gastric bypass surgery. While she initially did lose weight, one year later she was right back to her presurgery weight. Feeling like she was out of options, she eventually joined my class.

As Carly began sharing her story, it was clear that her negative body beliefs had been controlling her. For years she had been sitting on the sidelines, unwilling to participate in her own life, refusing to swim with her own kids even though she had always loved to swim. Since it involved wearing a bathing suit, she'd decided years ago that swimming was out of the question until she lost the weight.

One day, by tapping on her negative belief that there was nothing she could appreciate about her body, Carly experienced a huge and sudden shift. Before even losing a pound, she shared that for the first time in her adult life, she felt real love and gratitude for her body. "It's done so much for me," she explained. Soon afterward, Carly bought a bathing suit and went swimming with her children. Before tapping this hadn't felt like a possibility; even the thought of it terrified her.

A few days after she and I had tapped together on these beliefs, she sent me an e-mail. She wrote, "I feel amazing and brave! I cried because of all the joy I feel. Thank you."

Since changing her belief, she has spent several days at the pool swimming with her children and is excited about living a much more active life. Last I knew, she had signed up for a 5k race with her sister and had cut her hair short, after years of dreaming about it but never daring to do it.

How often do we put our lives on hold because of our own judgments and insecurities? That pool was always there; that joy was always there. It simply came down to Carly believing that she deserved

> Everybody has a part of their body that she doesn't like, but I've stopped complaining about mine because I don't want to critique nature's handiwork . . . My job is simply to allow the light to shine out of the masterpiece.
>
> —ALFRE WOODARD

it right now, not just after losing weight. Her decision to experience life now made it easier for her to take other steps forward in her life.

Take a moment now to think about how your body beliefs may be affecting your life. Are they holding you back, not just in your body confidence and weight loss journey but in preventing you from truly living and enjoying your life?

Now that you've begun to discover some of the limiting beliefs that have shaped your story, it's time to begin tapping! The first step is to tap on a belief, and then once you can say that old belief without feeling triggered, you can incorporate powerful affirmations.

# How to Tap on a Belief

Begin by saying the belief out loud or in your head. For example, "Losing weight is an uphill battle," or "There's nothing to appreciate about my body."

Ask yourself, on a scale of 0 to 10—with 10 being that your belief feels totally true and 0 being that you barely feel it—*How true does that belief feel?* Give it a number, and then begin tapping as you're stating the belief. For example:

**Karate Chop:** Even though there is nothing to appreciate about my body, I love and accept myself. (*Repeat three times.*)

**Eyebrow:** There is nothing to love about my body . . .

**Side of Eye:** Not when it looks like this.

**Under Eye:** I notice everything that is wrong.

**Under Nose:** I feel like my body is working against me.

**Chin:** If only I had been born into a different body . . .

**Collarbone:** This feels so unfair.

**Under Arm:** There is nothing to love about my body . . .

**Top of Head:** This story I've been telling myself . . .

*When the intensity of your initial tapping target(s) is 5 or lower, you can move on to the positive.*

**Eyebrow:** My body has been doing so well . . .

**Side of Eye:** Under this harsh internal environment.

## Getting Specific

As we discussed in Chapter 2, you want to be as specific as possible when you're tapping. Here are some questions you can ask yourself as you're tapping on your beliefs:

*"Who taught me this belief?"*

*"When did I pick up this belief?"*

*"Where do I feel this belief in my body?"*

You can say your answers out loud or in your mind as you begin to tap.

**Under Eye:** It does so much for me every day without my thanking it.

**Under Nose:** My body does everything to survive.

**Chin:** Now I give my body the love and support to thrive.

**Collarbone:** I create a nurturing internal environment.

**Under Arm:** My body is beautiful.

**Top of Head:** I'm grateful for my body.

*Take a deep breath and check in with how you feel. Measure the intensity again and continue tapping until you experience relief.*

## The Real Proof that Negative Beliefs Are False

If our negative beliefs and feelings were congruent with who we really are, we would feel satisfied. Instead, the negative beliefs we have about ourselves, our bodies, and our world feel incredibly painful. That's because they don't feel *right*. They are jarring to our soul because they go against our truth.

When I first heard this idea presented by Carol Tuttle, author of *Remembering Wholeness*, whom I've also interviewed for our annual Tapping World Summit, I was struck by how true it felt.

Think about it. If you really were not good enough, if your weight really was your genes' fault, and weight loss was biologically impossible, you would be satisfied with those beliefs. You would find peace within those beliefs because they would be congruent with who you are. The fact that you are dissatisfied with your beliefs—and the reason that some of your beliefs cause you pain—is that they are not a reflection of who you really are. So don't judge or fear those painful feelings; they are simply a signal that you have veered away from your truth.

> Don't judge or fear those painful feelings; they are simply a signal that you have veered away from your truth.
>
> —JESSICA ORTNER

If and when you take this journey and do the tapping to clear your negative beliefs and emotions, a new story will appear, a story that feels true to who you really are. Within that new story, you will clearly see and feel what you never could before—that you *are* good enough, and you *are* worthy. You will see that you have an incredible amount of power to create the life you have always wanted, and that you don't have to suffer or deprive yourself to get there. While your weight loss journey will become far easier, what will amaze you even more is how different your entire life looks and feels.

That shift into a new story often happens while tapping, but we frequently don't realize its significance until much later, at the most unexpected moments. One client of mine noticed the shift one day while shopping with her husband. Having always hated her own reflection, she was surprised to notice herself in a mirror in a new light. "Wow, I look really beautiful," she said out loud. Her husband smiled, gave her a kiss, and said, "I know, honey. I've been telling you that for years." In all their years together, it was the first time she had really heard him—and the first time she'd actually *felt* beautiful. Her story about herself and what was possible in her life had been rewritten.

That's what happens when we allow ourselves to create new beliefs that feel authentic to who we really are, and it's what will happen for you when you do the same.

•

# Letting Go of Limiting Beliefs and Creating Empowering Ones

**Karate Chop:** Even though I've held on to beliefs that have held me back, I love and accept myself. (*Repeat three times.*)

**Eyebrow:** All these limiting beliefs . . .

**Side of Eye:** I thought they were facts.

**Under Eye:** Many of them have been passed down from my parents . . .

**Under Nose:** Or from my culture . . .

**Chin:** "If it's not hard, it's not worth it" . . .

**Collarbone:** "I'm just unlucky" . . .

**Under Arm:** "I have bad genes" . . .

**Top of Head:** "I don't follow through" . . .

**Eyebrow:** These old beliefs . . .

**Side of Eye:** I've been repeating them to myself.

**Under Eye:** These beliefs don't have power.

**Under Nose:** I've been giving them power with my attention.

**Chin:** I allow myself to question everything.

**Collarbone:** Is this really true?

**Under Arm:** Is this really what I believe?

**Top of Head:** I stay open and curious.

**Eyebrow:** I logically know they aren't true . . .

**Side of Eye:** But they feel true.

**Under Eye:** Acknowledging this feeling . . .

**Under Nose:** I've lived with them for so long.

**Chin:** I thought it was just who I was . . .

**Collarbone:** But it's a feeling . . .

**Under Arm:** And feelings can change.

**Top of Head:** I accept myself even with all these feelings.

**Eyebrow:** When I take time to notice these beliefs . . .

**Side of Eye:** I tap on them individually.

**Under Eye:** I have the power to choose what I believe.

**Under Nose:** If that old belief creeps up . . .

**Chin:** I tap on the emotion this old belief elicits.

**Collarbone:** I feel calm and confident . . .

**Under Arm:** I remember it's just a thought.

**Top of Head:** And then I choose a different thought.

**Eyebrow:** I consciously choose what I believe.

**Side of Eye:** I believe being healthy is empowering.

**Under Eye:** Life is meant to be enjoyed.

**Under Nose:** Health is an expression of that joy.

**Chin:** I can achieve my goals.

**Collarbone:** My body is supporting me.

**Under Arm:** I have so much to be grateful for.

**Top of Head:** I possess every quality needed to live an extraordinary life.

Fill in the last round yourself! What do you now choose to believe about yourself?

I am . . .
Adventurous
Confident
Determined
Enough
Intelligent
Passionate
Smart
Strong
Unstoppable
Worthy

**Eyebrow:** I am _____

**Side of Eye:** I am _____

**Under Eye:** I am _____

**Under Nose:** I am _____

**Chin:** I am _____

**Collarbone:** I am _____

**Under Arm:** I am _____

**Top of Head:** I am _____

# Chapter 7

# The Pain Beneath the Weight

One of the hardest things to understand when we're struggling with weight is that weight is a symptom; it's not the actual problem. When I say this to clients, they immediately counter with something like "But I can't be happy because of my weight" or "I can't go to my high school reunion because of my weight" or "I can't get a date or have a relationship because of my weight."

Seeing weight as the problem is a logical conclusion, a belief that many of us have used to protect ourselves from the true meaning of the weight. When we dig deeper, we discover that it's the pain beneath the weight that prevents us from losing weight and feeling confident in the body we have. Often, we find that the weight has been protecting us, making us feel safe on some level. When we're able to process the pain beneath the weight, we can finally release this need for safety through weight. Only then can we wake up to our true potential and begin not just losing weight but living the life of our dreams.

Before you explore the pain beneath the weight, however, you first need to step back and take a look at your relationship with your body.

## Even if You Don't Love Your Body, Your Body Loves You

We've all experienced that excruciating moment when a paper cut first appears. What we often don't realize is how quickly the body goes to work to help us heal from it. Even before we shake our hand in pain, the blood vessels leading to the wound tighten to reduce blood flow to the injured area; platelets quickly gather to form a plug; clotting proteins then join in to stop the bleeding. For weeks afterward, the body works around the clock to complete the injury recovery process.

> Your physical body loves you unconditionally. Even if you judge your body, even if you reject it and don't like it, your body is completely loyal to you.
>
> —DON MIGUEL RUIZ

How often do we feel grateful for all that the body is doing for us? For many, the answer is never.

Most of us have spent so much time and energy judging and criticizing the body we have that we've forgotten to notice how hard it works to support us. The reason tapping is such a powerful healing modality is that it releases the stress that interferes with the body's ability to do what it was designed to do—recover and heal. The challenge is that when we have unconscious programs that teach us it's not safe to let go of the weight, the body will follow the mind's signals and hold on to weight in an attempt to protect itself.

## Your Body, Your Weight, and Your Safety

When we look at the body and the unconscious mind's primal instinct to keep us safe, we often overlook the possibility that holding on to extra weight can be one way in which the body is trying to protect us. Jon Gabriel lost 220 pounds by first addressing the underlying emotions that were causing his body to hold on to weight. In *The Gabriel Method* he describes this connection:

If you are currently carrying extra weight, then your body believes it is not safe to lose weight; it is fighting for your life. When your body believes that it is safe to lose weight—or better, safer to be thin—your body will *force* you to lose weight. You will be working with your body's natural laws instead of violating them. Weight loss will then become automatic, effortless, and inevitable.

Since publishing his book, Gabriel has explained how tapping contributes to this process:

At least 80 percent of the people I work with who are overweight have emotional or past trauma challenges contributing to their weight gain. Tapping is one of the simplest, most effective tools anyone can use to immediately start seeing results.

To look more closely at how weight may be keeping you safe, let's explore some of the issues that may make your unconscious mind see weight as a source of safety—and conversely, weight loss as a threat.

## When Weight Protects You from a Person or Relationship

Weight often acts as a physical barrier between us and some person or group that makes us feel unsafe. That was the pattern Carol discovered with her own weight. For years her job had required her to move to a new city within the U.S. every few years. She made an interesting connection: she realized that the closer she moved to her mother, the more weight she gained.

Carol's mother was what she called an "energy vampire." Through tapping, Carol realized that she didn't need to focus on her weight but instead needed to tap on her anger toward her mother. Her body had been using weight as a protective barrier, a way to keep Carol from being drained emotionally by her mother.

## When Losing Weight Feels Unsafe

As we've discussed in previous chapters, repeatedly asking ourselves what the secondary gain of our weight is, and looking at this in different contexts, is an important part of the weight loss and body confidence journey. We often don't realize how weight is serving us, allowing us to avoid emotional pain that we're not comfortable facing. While on a conscious level we feel desperate to lose the weight, when we tap on what feels scary about losing weight, we're often surprised by what we discover.

By clearing her anger with tapping, Carol began to feel strong enough to say no to her mother. It was a huge breakthrough. By liberating herself from her mother's controlling energy, she realized she no longer needed or wanted to use food to numb her feelings toward her mother. She also didn't need the weight to shield her from her mother.

Ask yourself: *Is there a relationship in my life that I feel I need protection from?* If so, how does that relationship make you feel? Give that feeling a number on the scale of 0 to 10, and then begin tapping.

Even though this relationship with _____ makes me feel _____, I love and accept myself and choose to stand strong in my power.

## When Weight Protects You from Facing Important Challenges

It was her marriage, not her weight, that most needed Tara's attention. She was terrified that losing weight would give her enough confidence to leave her husband, and she felt overwhelmed by the idea of starting over. Having already been through one divorce, she didn't want to go through another one.

When Tara focused her daily tapping on the sadness she felt around the state of her marriage, she realized that she wasn't willing to give up on it. The weight, she quickly saw, was just her body's way of getting her attention. Once she took action and began to focus on repairing and rebuilding her marriage, the weight seemed to fall off. She lost 16 pounds in two months and ended up at the exact weight she had been when she married her husband.

Take a moment to ask yourself: "If I wasn't busy obsessing about my weight, what would I have to face? What emotions do I feel when I think about that part of my life?" Feel free to write them down and rate the intensity on a scale of 0 to 10. Try beginning your tapping with the setup statement "Even though I'm scared to face this . . . I love and accept myself and I am safe . . . " Repeat it three times while tapping on the karate chop point, and get more specific about your tapping target as you tap.

**Eyebrow:** This thing I don't want to face . . .

**Side of Eye:** I don't feel like I can handle it.

**Under Eye:** I would be overwhelmed . . .

**Under Nose:** So I ignore it . . .

**Chin:** By blaming my body.

**Collarbone:** This area in my life . . .

**Under Arm:** That I don't want to see . . .

**Top of Head:** It feels like too much.

*When the intensity of your initial tapping target(s) is 5 or lower, you can move on to the positive.*

**Eyebrow:** I have everything within me now . . .

**Side of Eye:** To address this area in my life with love.

**Under Eye:** I don't need to find the solution . . .

**Under Nose:** I just need to seek the first step.

**Chin:** I take this one step at a time.

**Collarbone:** It is safe for me to face these emotions.

**Under Arm:** I have patience with this process . . .

**Top of Head:** And faith in my abilities.

*Take a deep breath and check in with how you feel. Measure the intensity again and continue tapping until you experience relief.*

## When Weight Is a Form of Self-Punishment

Sometimes we find that we're bingeing and holding on to weight in order to punish ourselves. That was the case for Lena, who discovered that the weight was a way of punishing herself for a painful decision she had made years before.

While living with her former partner in his native homeland several years ago, she had been shocked to watch him transform from a kind and loving partner into a physically and verbally abusive tyrant. Just as she was trying to digest the change in his character, Lena learned that she was pregnant. During that same time, a violent civil war broke out in the country where they were living. People were being shot down daily in the streets near where they lived, and she began feeling increasingly desperate to return to her own home several thousand miles away. Terrified that her abusive partner would make her stay if he learned of her pregnancy, Lena was equally terrified by the idea of having a baby in the midst of war and subjecting her baby to an abusive father.

Lena felt alone and heartbroken by the turn her relationship and her life had taken, and she felt she had no choice but to have an abortion. She was deeply ashamed of her decision and told no one about it. Although it had seemed at the time to be her only real option, as time went on she felt that she, too, had died that day. How could she deserve to live after she had ended another life?

Soon after returning to her home, Lena was diagnosed with chronic fatigue syndrome and quickly began gaining weight. As we tapped on the memories, emotions, and beliefs she had been carrying around since the abortion, she was finally able to let herself grieve the loss of her baby. She sobbed as she processed her emotions while tapping, giving a voice to the shame and pain she had been carrying around for so many years.

During our tapping session, Lena realized that the best way to honor her baby's lost life was to live her own. For the first time since the abortion, she could see herself as a good and loving person who had done her best under very painful circumstances. "I felt such an enormous relief as you helped me accept and own my choice and send the memory of the baby to the light. I have finally forgiven myself," she shared in an e-mail shortly after the session.

Weeks later, I was thrilled to get another e-mail from her saying that since our session, she'd shared the story of her abortion with three close friends. Before tapping on it, she'd felt too ashamed to tell anyone about her baby. Because she had been able to give a voice to the past while tapping, she had calmed the panic in her body. Once calm, she could tell the story while feeling compassion toward herself. That made it easier to reach out and get support from people who loved and respected her. This is an important breakthrough because when we feel shame around a certain experience, we often feel we need to hide the pain, punish ourselves, and suffer in silence. We are scared that others will judge us the way we harshly judge ourselves. When we begin to show compassion toward ourselves, we attract people with compassionate hearts and discover that we are not alone.

I share this story not to judge or ignite political or religious debate but because I've worked with many women like Lena who have been walking around secretly mourning the loss of their babies, feeling utterly alone and unable to reach out for support. When they have nowhere to turn, their bodies accumulate weight, hoping to protect them from the emotional pain they've felt since having an abortion.

Once they're able to process the emotions they have been holding in, their bodies become willing and able to release the weight. More important, they finally stop blaming themselves for what was often a very painful decision.

Whether it's an abortion or another difficult decision we have made in our lives, the world needs us to forgive ourselves. We may look back and wish we'd made a different choice, but until we can see that we were doing our best in that moment, we remain stuck in the past, unable to evolve beyond it.

How many women are not lighting up the world because of the pain they feel from a past event? We feel we need to punish ourselves, but self-punishment only adds to our pain.

Whatever issues or memories may be holding you back and causing your body to seek extra weight for protection, I urge you to speak your secret and do tapping on it. Take a moment now to ask yourself, *What am I using weight to protect myself from?* Write down your answer on a piece of paper, if you'd like.

## From Self-Punishment to Self-Acceptance

In middle school after being caught cheating on a math test, I went to my dad and asked what my punishment was. I remember feeling like I wanted and needed to be punished, so I was stunned when he said there would be no punishment. Confused, I asked him why not, and he replied, "Because I know how hard you are on yourself. Nothing I could do could punish you the way you punish yourself." I was blessed with incredibly kind parents who weren't happy with me cheating on a math test but who also wanted me to be able to love myself. I don't know where I picked up the habit of self-punishment, but even when I was a preteen my parents recognized it. Somewhere I picked up the belief that I wasn't good enough, and I thought that if I punished myself enough, maybe I would be forgiven by a man with a white beard in the sky. I believed that punishing myself and being hard on myself made me a good person.

So many women I work with take secret pride in how much they punish themselves over things both big and small. Because they don't feel they deserve happiness, they feel justified in their cruelty toward themselves. Their bodies then respond by holding on to weight, hoping to somehow stay safe inside the harsh internal environment they have created.

It's time to release our pain, learn to forgive ourselves, and realize that self-punishment isn't the answer; self-love and self-acceptance are.

> We achieve inner health only through forgiveness—the forgiveness not only of others but also of ourselves.
>
> —JOSHUA LOTH LIEBMAN

Let's do some tapping now on forgiving ourselves. Pick an event that you feel you need to punish yourself for and rate its emotional intensity on a scale of 0 to 10. Keep it in your mind as you tap.

**Karate Chop:** Even though I feel I should punish myself, I love, accept, and forgive myself. (*Repeat three times.*)

**Eyebrow:** This thing that happened . . .

**Side of Eye:** I feel so ashamed.

**Under Eye:** I can't change what happened.

**Under Nose:** It all feels hopeless . . .

**Chin:** So instead I punish myself.

**Collarbone:** Somewhere I learned . . .

**Under Arm:** In order to be "good" I need to punish myself . . .

**Top of Head:** But no good is coming from this punishment.

*When the intensity of your initial tapping target is 5 or lower, you can move on to the positive.*

**Eyebrow:** I can only face darkness with light.

**Side of Eye:** I choose to bring a new light to this situation.

**Under Eye:** What happened isn't a reflection of who I am.

**Under Nose:** I express who I really am right now by choosing love and compassion.

**Chin:** I was doing the best I could at the time.

**Collarbone:** I have learned so much, and I choose a new path.

**Under Arm:** I love, accept, and forgive myself.

**Top of Head:** My future is bright.

*Take a deep breath and check in with how you feel. Measure the intensity again and continue tapping until you experience relief.*

## When Weight Is Your Best Excuse

When we've been struggling with weight for years, it can become our best excuse for not pursuing our dreams or facing our fears.

Finish this sentence for yourself by filling in the blank: I can't _____ because of the weight.

How you complete that sentence gives you insight into what's going on below the surface that's causing you to hold on to the weight.

In her 40s and two years after her divorce, Michelle insisted that she couldn't date until she lost weight. She would look at herself in the mirror and think, *Who would want to love this?* She resented her body because she felt like it stopped her from the one thing she longed to have in her life—romance.

Knowing that the body is always protecting us, I asked her to imagine losing the weight and then walking into a restaurant and sitting across from a potential partner. "How does that image make you feel?" I asked. She was surprised to realize how panicked she felt by the thought of dating. Opening herself up to love and romance might mean reliving the pain she had experienced with her ex-husband, and that terrified her. We began tapping on her fear while focusing on memories from her marriage that still triggered her emotionally. After that session and before losing a pound, Michelle began to date successfully. She realized that it hadn't been her weight stopping her, but her fear.

When I first began to tap on my weight, I filled in the blank with "I can't be successful." As someone in the health and wellness industry, I felt like I needed to be "perfect" in order to help others. Although I loved interviewing people, I would shy away from

> Do nothing, say nothing, and be nothing, and you'll never be criticized.
>
> —ELBERT HUBBARD

the camera because I didn't feel pretty enough. When I dug deeper, I realized that my real fears were of being judged. If I didn't do anything, no one else could judge me. (That same fear is often why people don't finish a project. If it's not finished, it can't be critiqued. If a book is never finished, it can never be negatively reviewed.)

As I continued tapping, I realized that I was actually afraid of criticism that had already happened. The more I tapped on times when I'd been judged, the more I understood that the things people say about me (or anyone) are a reflection of their own beliefs about themselves.

Soon after, we hosted our annual Tapping World Summit, and during that event my new awareness was put to the test. One weekend morning during that summit, someone posted a mean comment about me on my Facebook page. Later that day while at brunch with some girlfriends, I announced that I had my first hater. One of my friends jumped up and said, "Cheers to haters! If you don't have them, it means you're not doing anything worthwhile." We all laughed.

To be our true authentic selves, we eventually have to rock the boat. As we'll see next, what often happens is that our fear of shining overshadows all else and threatens to rob us of the happiness, success, and love we so deserve.

## Tapping on What You Think People Would Say

In my work with thousands of women, I've found that imaginary dialogues in which we are criticized by others are incredibly common. Often what we fear we'll hear from others has never been uttered. The reason it feels so real is because it's an inner reflection of our own beliefs and fears. By tapping on what we think someone would say to us, we're often able to build even stronger relationships with that person. At other times, tapping on this helps us realize that we have allowed a toxic person or group of people into our lives. Instead of creating a boundary by holding on to weight, we can then create an energetic boundary and allow ourselves to spend less time with that person or group.

Take a moment now to ask yourself, *What negative feedback am I afraid I'll get if I'm successful at losing the weight?* Feel free to write down the words and phrases you think people would say. Be as specific as possible, including pinpointing who you think might say these things to you. Then say those words or phrases out loud while you tap through the points.

## Why Isn't It Safe for You to Shine?

Throughout her childhood, Ellie's success in school and with her art had always gotten a lot of attention, but it pained her that the praise she received seemed to detract from others. She feared that her success would make other people judge both her and themselves negatively. As a result, Ellie learned to deflect praise at a young age.

She also had the habit of comparing herself to other women and feeling "less than." Since she knew how bad this felt, she feared that if she were praised others would feel the same way. In order to avoid that, she downplayed any successes and shrank away from compliments.

As an adult, Ellie felt very uncomfortable being noticed, especially for the art that had always been her true calling and passion. Occasionally, when the urge to create got too overwhelming, she would release something only to shrink away as soon as her art received positive attention, which it often did. As the years passed and she worked harder and harder at playing small to avoid attention, Ellie gained weight and increasingly resented her body.

During my class, Ellie realized that it wasn't her weight that she needed to tap on but all of the issues related to her fear of shining. After tapping, however, she could see that shining her light was a gift, not a burden. Soon afterward she began to share her art for the first time in many years.

After having that breakthrough, she posted this painting about how much pain we experience when we constantly compare ourselves to others in our private Weight Loss & Body Confidence online student community.

I was so in love with it that I shared it on my fan page and reached out to Ellie to let her know how much I loved her work. I then asked her if she would contribute artwork to this book. By clearing her fear of shining, Ellie had the courage to share her art and enrich all of our lives. She was also able to get her art published for the first time ever.

Without her focusing on it, Ellie's relationship with food also began to change. After years of trying to break her addiction to soda, within that

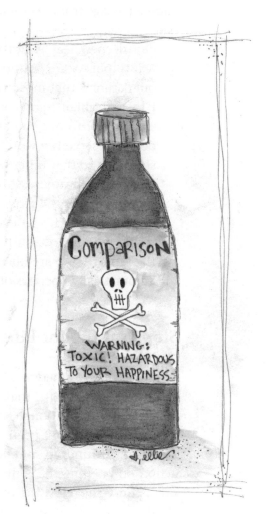

first month of tapping she was amazed when her soda cravings simply faded away. By allowing herself to shine with her art and throughout her life, she also began to feel calm and in control around food for the first time in years.

So many women I work with are so afraid to shine that they become desperate to deny their own potential and downplay their accomplishments. They're trying to play so small that they almost force themselves to use their weight to hide.

When it comes to our fear of shining, Marianne Williamson's oft-quoted passage from *Return to Love* says it best:

> Our deepest fear is not that we are inadequate. Our deepest fear is that we are powerful beyond measure. It is our light, not our darkness that most frightens us. We ask ourselves, Who am I to be brilliant, gorgeous, talented, fabulous? Actually, who are you *not* to be? You are a child of God. Your playing small does not serve the world. There is nothing enlightened about shrinking so that other people won't feel insecure around you. We are all meant to shine, as children do. We were born to make manifest the glory of God that is within us. It's not just in some of us; it's in everyone. And as we let our own light shine, we unconsciously give other people permission to do the same. As we are liberated from our own fear, our presence automatically liberates others.

## Stop Waiting for Life to Begin

Whatever you're afraid to do but really want to do is exactly what you need to do. For Leigh, that meant realizing her dream of opening a wellness center. Although she'd owned the property for more than four years, she hadn't been able to motivate herself to make the contacts, get the funding, and do the marketing she needed to do. Taking action on opening the center was yet another project she would take on . . . once she'd lost the weight.

When Leigh began tapping on her fear of shining, she realized that it was a lack of self-love, not the need for weight loss, that was preventing her from opening her wellness center. She had been told since childhood that she needed to "be quiet" and "stop talking," and it didn't feel safe for her to shine. For that reason, her dream of opening a wellness center felt terrifying.

Armed with that new self-awareness, Leigh began tapping daily on her fear of shining, using my tapping meditation on that topic. Within a few weeks' time she made more progress on opening her wellness center than she had in years. Suddenly she began making contacts and hearing from people who wanted to support her efforts, including a woman who offered to donate her time to create a website for the center. Leigh was amazed and thrilled by the outpouring of support and interest.

> Life shrinks or expands in proportion to one's courage.
>
> —ANAÏS NIN

During those same few weeks, Leigh also began planning healthy meals and exercising regularly. Suddenly these lifestyle changes felt easy and enjoyable. The weight and inches began falling off almost immediately. What made her really smile, though, was that before she'd even lost all the weight she'd originally intended to lose, she could pass by a mirror and appreciate her body for the first time in years.

Several weeks after the class ended, she shared this with me:

I'm down 11 pounds and have definitely stepped into my shine! I'm watching my body and behaviors change daily. I'm no longer emotionally eating on a daily basis, and I love and embrace exercise. I can walk by the mirror without insulting myself . . . all really big things for me. Every day I still continue to learn and evolve, and that's the fun part! I know I get better every day. Tapping has been a real game changer. And I still do the meditations . . . I love them.

## Stepping into Your Best Self and Biggest Dreams

People often ask me how I incorporate tapping into my daily life. Here is an exercise I do every night.

First, visualize what you most desire, beginning by focusing on just one thing. It might be a desire to feel strong and confident in your body, to share a gift or talent, to speak up, or to be in a more loving relationship. Magnify that image in your mind. Breathe deeply and really feel what it feels like to be in that space. Then ask yourself, *Does anything feel uncomfortable about this image? Can I feel comfortable in my body when I see this image in my mind?* If you feel your stomach or shoulders clenching, for example, that is an indication that this image is creating stress in your body. Continue breathing deeply while tapping through the points and focusing on the image. If any specific fears or other negative emotions or self-talk come up, keep tapping through the points while you visualize what you desire. Keep doing this until you can visualize this desire while feeling calm and congruent in your body.

This is an incredibly powerful exercise to use on a regular basis. You'll find that your dreams will continue to expand as your comfort zone grows.

## Being Afraid, Overwhelmed, and More—It's All Normal

When we start looking at how the weight has been keeping us safe, and how we can release that need and then begin to let ourselves shine, we may feel hints of excitement. Often, though, we're quickly overcome by fear. It's normal to feel afraid and overwhelmed. The key is to learn from these feelings but not be controlled by them. That's where tapping comes in. Tapping on our emotions doesn't mean we'll never feel fear and other negative emotions again. Tapping is a tool that helps us maneuver through emotions so we can move forward in spite of the normal and natural emotional resistance we may experience.

At times when we look at how to let ourselves shine, part of feeling overwhelmed and afraid may come from not knowing what we're meant to do, or not knowing how to realize our dreams. That's also normal. By tapping on these emotions, we can reconnect with our intuition and through that, get clearer on our answers to these questions.

When you think about your dream, how overwhelmed do you feel on a scale of 0 to 10? Are there any other emotions or negative beliefs that grab your attention? Do you feel any tension in your body? Use the answers to these questions to help you be specific.

Let's do some tapping now:

**Karate Chop:** Even though I feel overwhelmed by this dream, I love and accept myself. (*Repeat three times.*)

**Eyebrow:** I feel so overwhelmed.

**Side of Eye:** There is so much to do.

**Under Eye:** I don't even know where to start.

**Under Nose:** What if I can't do this?

**Chin:** What if I make a mistake?

**Collarbone:** What if something goes wrong?

**Under Arm:** All these fears around pursuing this dream . . .

**Top of Head:** I give them a voice now.

*When the intensity of your initial tapping target is 5 or lower, you can move on to the positive.*

**Eyebrow:** Maybe I don't need to know every answer.

**Side of Eye:** Maybe I don't need to know exactly how I'll get there.

**Under Eye:** I focus on the single step ahead of me.

**Under Nose:** It's safe to take this step . . .

**Chin:** And trust that the answers will appear.

**Collarbone:** I can enjoy this process.

**Under Arm:** It feels so good to take this step forward.

**Top of Head:** It's safe for me to step up.

*Take a deep breath and check in with how you feel. Measure the intensity again and continue tapping until you experience relief.*

What action can you take right now toward a dream? Maybe it's simply writing an e-mail or making a phone call. Trust your intuition and take a step forward, no matter how small that step may seem.

## The Time Between Now and Later Is Called Life—Don't Miss It!

After participating in my class and doing the tapping, Brandy was feeling happy in her skin for the first time in many years. One day while riffling through a shoebox full of old photos, she came across a picture of herself wearing a green bikini when she was in her early 30s. As she looked at the beautiful woman in the picture, she remembered hating her body at the moment the picture was taken.

As she thought back to that moment, she felt compassion for the woman in the picture who couldn't recognize her own beauty. She was heavier now, yet she felt more beautiful than she had when that picture was taken because she had been tapping on her beliefs about herself.

The following weekend Brandy went camping with her husband. As she put on her bathing suit, her old critical voice began creeping in. As soon as she heard it, she smiled. That voice no longer controlled her. She realized that if she didn't enjoy her life and body now, she would be wasting even more opportunities for joy, just as she had missed the opportunity to feel good in her green bikini all those years ago.

It's important to have goals and reach for your dreams, but it's never a reason not to enjoy the present moment. Ultimately it's the journey, not the result, that brings the most happiness.

It's time, right this second, to stop and smell the roses. Notice the parts of your body that are beautiful. Notice how you feel when you take a moment to place your hand on your heart and take a deep breath.

Living a fabulous life means recognizing how fabulous you and your life are right now.

## Feeling Safe to Shine

**Karate Chop:** Even though it doesn't feel safe to shine, I love and accept myself. (*Repeat three times.*)

**Eyebrow:** It doesn't feel safe to shine.

**Side of Eye:** It doesn't feel safe to try my best.

**Under Eye:** I might get too much attention.

**Under Nose:** Someone else might not like it.

**Chin:** It's safer to play small behind a bigger body.

**Collarbone:** Part of me wants to shine and be my best . . .

**Under Arm:** Part of me doesn't feel it's safe.

**Top of Head:** This inner struggle . . .

**Eyebrow:** I've been battling with myself.

**Side of Eye:** It feels safer to stay the same.

**Under Eye:** It doesn't feel safe to lose weight.

**Under Nose:** It doesn't feel safe to feel confident now . . .

**Chin:** Because I had a negative reaction in the past.

**Collarbone:** I give those feelings a voice now . . .

**Under Arm:** And let them go.

**Top of Head:** I've learned so much since then.

**Eyebrow:** Somewhere I learned it wasn't safe to shine . . .

**Side of Eye:** This old belief that's held me back.

**Under Eye:** What they said and how they reacted . . .

**Under Nose:** Was a reflection on them, not me.

**Chin:** I acknowledge how it made me feel.

**Collarbone:** I've feared another negative reaction . . .

**Under Arm:** So it's better to surrender to fear and play small.

**Top of Head:** But I want more.

**Eyebrow:** I have a choice to make.

**Side of Eye:** I can care what everyone else thinks . . .

**Under Eye:** At the expense of my happiness . . .

**Under Nose:** Or care what I think . . .

**Chin:** And shine brightly.

**Collarbone:** I have courage and faith . . .

**Under Arm:** I choose to shine.

**Top of Head:** I inspire others to do the same.

**Eyebrow:** I feel the relief of letting myself shine.

**Side of Eye:** Holding myself back was exhausting . . .

**Under Eye:** I allow my imagination to run free.

**Under Nose:** I'm pulled forward toward my dreams . . .

**Chin:** I surrender to the voice in my heart.

**Collarbone:** I know what to do . . .

**Under Arm:** And I can take action now.

**Top of Head:** It's safe for me to shine.

# Chapter 8

# Feeling Confident in Your Feminine Body

From a young age we are bombarded with images and ideals about our own sexuality and femininity. We must be sexy, society suggests, but never slutty. We must be beautiful but not too confident; not prudish, but not promiscuous, either. Too often, we're thrown into our sexuality before we're ready to acknowledge and understand it. Then, just when we begin to celebrate our new and ever-changing bodies, we're faced with unwanted sexual attention and sometimes even blamed and shamed for provoking it.

Society places so many conflicting beliefs and expectations on us that our relationship with our own sexuality seems doomed from the start. After being subjected to our culture's angst around female sexuality, many of us unconsciously look to weight as a way to hide from sexual attention that has felt, and often still feels, confusing and threatening.

Next we'll explore how our relationship with our sexuality has impacted us and our weight, and discover new ways of relating to our bodies and our power that allows us to experience a much longed for feeling of freedom.

As we'll see next, for many of us, this tortured relationship with our sexuality begins with puberty, just as we're beginning to get breasts.

## Being a Girl in a Woman's Body

I grew up a tomboy, refusing to wear a dress even when it meant I had to have another shouting match with my mom. If my brothers didn't have to wear dresses, neither did I. Wanting so badly to be just like them, I did everything possible to act like a boy. I was a rebel, outspoken, and rarely shy, forever eager for the next adventure. Most of my childhood summers I spent running around the woods with my many guy friends.

Then suddenly, my breasts arrived and ruined it all. One guy friend admitted that some boys were referring to me as "the girl with boobs" and making jokes behind my back. I hated my body for betraying me, bringing me all this teasing and weird attention.

Unable to make sense of it all, I used food to cope with my anxiety. Hiding behind weight wasn't a conscious decision, but it served me well, protecting me from being objectified and isolated long before I was ready for it.

This pattern of beginning to hide from our newly sensual bodies the moment they start to develop is one I've seen repeatedly in clients. Although puberty may seem like a distant memory, those early years of feeling like a little girl suddenly inhabiting a womanly body can have a lasting impact on our relationship with our femininity and weight.

One student, Laura, traced her relationship with her body and weight back to when she was first teased on the school bus for her newly growing breasts. Embarrassed and ashamed, she began wearing a poncho that her grandmother had knitted for her. No matter what the weather was, that poncho was her favorite way to hide her feminine body. As she grew older, whenever she lost weight she felt uncomfortable with any attention she might receive, whether it was from men or a friend commenting about how great she looked. Her early experiences in school had led her to associate having a feminine form with being a target of teasing and unwanted attention.

For so many of us, puberty came as a shock. Unprepared for breasts, menstruation, and the new curves that began appearing in the mirror, we blamed the body for changes that seemed uncomfortable and unsafe.

Take a moment to think back on how puberty felt to you. Are there any events or memories around puberty that taught you it wasn't safe to be in a woman's body? If so, tell the story while you tap now. Feel free to refer back to Chapter 5, where we learned how to tap through past events.

## Compliments: An Unexpected Trigger

When we haven't been taught how to create a positive relationship with our femininity and sexuality, any kind of attention, including compliments, can feel profoundly unsettling. While that may seem counterintuitive at first, when we lack body confidence and have struggled with weight, we often fear any kind of attention because it could lead to us being hurt or humiliated again.

That was the case for Lori, who had lost 18 pounds while taking my class. She had been working on her fear of shining and realized she had stopped wearing the oversized gray jacket that she used to wear all the time, regardless of the weather. Finally feeling confident and ready to leave the "gray" behind, one day she decided to wear a white sweater with a pair of pants she hadn't been able to fit into for a few years. When she left the house she felt incredible—beautiful, radiant, and full of energy.

She was running errands later that day when a man whistled at her and muttered, "Ooh, sexy lady." Feeling threatened by his comment, her whole body immediately became tense. Her panic was so acute that she froze. Unable to speak and unsure how to react, she looked down and quickly walked into a store. Part of her felt disgusted by this man, violated by his comment, but another part of her felt flattered that she, a married woman in her 50s, could still attract attention. When she realized this, she began to feel guilty for feeling flattered. Later that evening Lori still felt the burn of his comment, overwhelmed by feelings of shame and confusion.

Lori reached out to me a couple of weeks later, sharing that she was amazed that a single comment from a random stranger had derailed her entire day. It's a common occurrence when we don't allow our-selves to create boundaries with people, which is a topic we'll continue to explore throughout this chapter.

Lori and I tapped on the man's comment together, and she began to ground herself in her body and own her power. She repeated what he had said out loud, focused on the anxiety she felt in her body, and simply tapped while giving those feelings a voice. As she released her panicked response to the man's sexual attention, she could remember the comment without feeling threatened by it. By the end of our ses-sion, she imagined herself in that same situation but this time feeling present and confident in her body. After tapping through her shame and fear, she realized that she was in control and able to feel strong and powerful. When we feel panic around unsolicited attention, it's often because we feel powerless over the situation or unable to protect ourselves. One comment can lead us to feel frozen and powerless. It's helpful to understand why we freeze.

## The Freeze Response

Although Lori didn't freeze physically, she felt emotionally and men-tally frozen. The freeze response can take many forms, including feel-ing physically tense or frozen; holding your breath; agreeing when you disagree; or feeling unable to say no, speak up, or remove yourself from a situation. We see the physical manifestation of this freeze response in animals that live in the wild. When they are attacked, their bodies go stiff, and at a quick glance they don't appear to be breathing. This is where the phrase "playing possum" comes from, since the freeze response has been well documented in possums.

Because most predators are only interested in killing prey that fights back and won't eat an animal until they have killed it, the freeze response can be a powerful way for animals to protect themselves. When the attacker has lost interest in its unmoving body, the animal comes out of the freeze response and runs to safety.

Although we often use the fact that we froze to blame ourselves for not doing or saying more, in fact, the freeze response is our body's most primal way of protecting us. It's important to know this so we don't judge ourselves for freezing.

When we have experienced the freeze response in the past, we often fear the future because we feel defenseless around anything and anyone that seems to threaten us, which can include all kinds of confrontations and conflicts. When we tap while focusing on the event where we froze and allow ourselves to really feel what we were feeling, we lessen our need to go into the freeze response in the future. As a result, we can stay grounded and make conscious decisions that serve us.

Let's now do some brief tapping on a time when you may have had a freeze response in the past. If you remember several times when you had this response, that's okay. Start with a memory that isn't very intense. Did you freeze when someone asked you to commit to a project you didn't want to, or treat you in a way you weren't comfortable with?

*Note*: If your freeze response was a reaction to an intense trauma, please seek professional help. It's important to have the support you need before exploring ways to overcome the trauma. A growing number of therapists are incorporating tapping into their practices.

## How We Interpret Compliments

Just like Lori, many clients tell me they don't like getting compliments in any form, especially from men. "When a guy whistles at me on the street, I look down and panic," they say. "I get grossed out and feel violated, like they're undressing me with their eyes. But then part of me likes the attention and that makes me feel guilty and ashamed."

Being flattered by a compliment does not mean you're "asking for it," and it certainly doesn't mean you're at risk of cheating on your partner or spouse. So often we don't just fear the person but our perceived inability to do anything. In reality, however, when we're grounded in the body we have more power than we previously imagined. When someone compliments you, the first thing to notice is your breathing.

If it feels shallow and strained, your body is most likely having a stress response. By tapping on the experience, you can more quickly return to a calm state.

When I used tapping to address my own stress response to compliments and attention, particularly from men, I naturally began reacting to men differently. While I no longer felt panicked by their attention, I also realized that I had gotten very used to feeling uncomfortable when a man complimented me. I began making a conscious effort to notice my reaction and feelings whenever I got attention and then tap on my experiences. Over time, I became able to receive compliments for what they most often are—well-meaning compliments. Instead of feeling threatened, I can now enjoy them or ignore them. Either way, I feel present and in control.

## Responding to Catcalls

Living in New York City, my friends and I often talk about how often men use "catcalls" to get our attention. One day, I e-mailed a few of them and asked how they respond to catcalls in ways that make them feel empowered rather than victimized.

One friend shared that she usually just smiles back, sometimes even laughs, not at them but with them, like "You guys are crazy, you know that?" That way, she says, it feels like it's a harmless little flirtation.

Another friend responded that sometimes she accepts catcalls as compliments, but when she doesn't get a good feeling she just walks faster and ignores them. The difference is that she can stay present in her body and judge each situation individually.

Unfortunately we can't control what other people say, but we do have control over how we react and feel. It's okay if you find all catcalls inappropriate. The key is to know that you have the power to feel calm and present in your body if you do hear them.

Just the other day I was trying to hail a taxi in New York City at the worst time of day, 4 P.M., the time when most taxi drivers' shifts turn over. I'd forgotten about that and needed to get somewhere quickly. A taxi pulled up and I climbed in. As soon as I was safely inside, the driver said, "My shift is over, but you look so good in that blue dress, I had to stop." Because I didn't feel threatened in that particular situation, I smiled, and said, "Well then, I'll have to remember to wear this dress every time I try to catch a cab at four!" We both laughed.

Before I tapped on my emotional and physical reactions to unwanted attention, I would have responded by feeling afraid, perhaps even clenching up physically, and then had thoughts like *What a sexist pig.* Or I might have felt consumed by anger at getting unsolicited attention. Instead, because I could remain present and calm, I could easily survey whether this felt like a dangerous situation and then act accordingly.

## When Any Attention Is Too Much Attention

Sometimes we can be triggered by compliments from people who aren't threatening. That happened to me one time when my great-uncle said, "You look like you've lost weight." I smiled and thanked him, but inside I screamed, *Can we please stop making my body a topic of family conversation?*

Many women sheepishly confess to hearing the words "You look like you lost weight" and thinking, *So you thought I was fat before?* When body image is a massive open wound, even the gentlest touch of a feather can burn. We can't control what others say, but when we heal that wound we can choose to appreciate the soft touch of that feather and enjoy it as a compliment or simply ignore it.

Let's do some tapping now around receiving compliments, starting with the setup statement: *Even if someone notices my weight loss, I choose to feel*

> When body image is a massive open wound, even the gentlest touch of a feather can burn.
>
> —JESSICA ORTNER

*centered and powerful in my body*. Keep tapping on your experience around receiving compliments and see what you can process and clear.

## Creating Healthy Boundaries

When we feel uncomfortable receiving attention, that's usually an indication that we haven't been taught how to create healthy boundaries. We all naturally have boundaries but unless we know them and enforce them, people can cross them without much effort. When they do, we feel powerless and unsafe. As a result, we often blame ourselves and may also turn to weight as a form of self-protection.

This was true for Claire. When I asked her when she began gaining weight, she remembered the exact moment. After she lost 20 pounds, a male friend began telling her how great she looked while moving his hand up her thigh. By doing that he crossed a boundary that Claire didn't know how to keep. When I asked her why she didn't tell him to take his hand off her thigh, she said she didn't want to offend him or "make a big deal out of nothing."

As women, we're often taught to be "good girls." Don't upset anyone, don't offend anyone, don't do anything or you'll make it worse, we're told. Scared that we might disappoint or upset someone, we often judge and blame ourselves. We ask ourselves questions like, *Am I overthinking this, or being overly emotional?* But that's not it at all. The problem lies in the fact that we've never been taught how to create healthy boundaries, and this allows others to mistreat us.

Establishing boundaries is an essential part of living a healthy life, but it's hard to know where your boundaries are when you're not present in your body. When you are present in your body, you can quickly notice the feelings and sensations you experience when a boundary has been crossed.

Whenever you feel uncomfortable or unsafe, the first step is to physically remove yourself from the situation. If it doesn't feel right, say no. "No" is a full sentence. You do not need to explain yourself.

It can be helpful to begin tapping while focusing on any fear you have around standing in your power and having a clear voice. Once you've tapped on that, here is a positive tapping script to help incorporate this new idea.

**Eyebrow:** What I feel is more important . . .

**Side of Eye:** Than what anyone else thinks.

**Under Eye:** I am aware of my boundaries . . .

**Under Nose:** And stand firm in my power.

**Chin:** I feel strong and protected . . .

**Collarbone:** By the power of my own voice . . .

**Under Arm:** By the power of my large presence . . .

**Top of Head:** I am present and in control.

**Eyebrow:** I am a powerful adult.

**Side of Eye:** If something feels uncomfortable, I take immediate action.

**Under Eye:** I listen to my inner voice.

**Under Nose:** I don't need to understand my feelings . . .

**Chin:** I simply trust them.

**Collarbone:** I feel safe and powerful.

**Under Arm:** I have a clear voice and a strong presence.

**Top of Head:** I feel calm and confident.

## Using Your Energy to Maintain Boundaries

As we learn how to be present in the body and then create healthy boundaries for ourselves, it's important to also look at how energy can help us maintain those boundaries, even when we get more attention than we'd like or in some other way feel uncomfortable.

When I work with women on using their energy to maintain healthy boundaries, they often recall times when they stared someone down or said something that caused another person to retreat in some way. These are all examples of how we can use our energy to maintain boundaries that help us feel safe.

I'm often reminded of this when I go for a run. It's always the small dogs that scare me. They'll often come running toward me while barking so loudly that I physically jump out of fright. The big dogs are often a lot calmer and usually don't scare me. I like to keep a visual of the little dogs in my mind sometimes to remind myself that, when I need to, I, too, can be as intimidating as those small dogs with the big barks.

### Your Instincts Are Always Your Best Barometer

Gavin de Becker, author of *The Gift of Fear*, says that unlike other living creatures, humans will sense danger but ignore their intuitive hunch that something's wrong. Instead, they will reason themselves out of it and go toward the danger they sense. For example, women will often get onto an elevator even when they get a creepy feeling about the person already in it.

If you ever get a feeling that something's not right, you *must* pay attention to it. Trust and follow your instincts first, and worry about other people's judgments, thoughts, and feelings later. If you sense something is off, even if you can't explain how or why, be your own mother bear and get yourself into a better environment as quickly as you can.

# Your Body and Love

When we've received attention for having a feminine form, we sometimes create the false belief that the female body must look a certain way to attract romantic love. This is another pressure that many women feel. So let's look at how true or false this is.

YourTango, a love and relationships website, polled more than 20,000 men to figure out what traits initially attract men to women. Was it 0 percent body fat? Nope. The first response was sexual chemistry, second was smile, third was kindness, and fourth was sense of humor. General body type was after all of those at fifth place on the list. Your humor and kindness mean more to men than your body type.

So what about the first-place response, sexual chemistry? What is it exactly? Chemistry is energy. Have you ever had the experience of meeting a man or a woman with strong feminine or masculine energy, and although he or she is physically attractive to you, the moment you get close and begin speaking to him or her, your attraction vanishes? The person might have only commented on the weather but you suddenly sense some kind of energy that turns you off.

What attracts us to people is that spark. We are attracted to their energy. Does this mean that people don't care about looks? Of course not. But it does mean that your energy is far more important than your looks. We often forget this because we've picked up the belief that we are only worthy of love if we look a certain way. As a result, when we don't feel beautiful we shrink to avoid rejection.

When I believed that only perfectly thin women attracted "good guys," I could always find examples of that being true. If I was rejected by a guy, I made it mean that I just wasn't pretty enough and then used that as another reason not to share my true and natural energy. As a result, I often attracted men who were shrinking from their own potential and weren't able to accept me as my true self or be loving and trusting partners. When I did occasionally take a chance and was rejected, I took that as *more* evidence that I wasn't good enough. It was an endless cycle that I had created by not allowing myself to feel beautiful and confident in my own body.

## Using Weight to Test Love

If you believe that your body type attracts love, you may gain weight or resist losing weight in an attempt to rebel against that belief. You may then think that if you lose weight and someone falls in love with you, it's only because of your body. By remaining overweight, you can test your partner to make sure they love you for who you are and not for your body.

This type of rebellion comes from the limiting belief that your body attracts love. It can be very destructive to current relationships or impact your ability to find a loving relationship. You can be loved for your mind, body, and spirit. It's important to make the journey of body confidence and weight loss about how you feel in your body and your desire to thrive. Refer to Chapter 6 to tap on this belief.

When we believe that beauty attracts love and that we're not beautiful enough to be worthy of love, we're also unable to receive the love and affection we so desperately want because we don't feel we are worthy. We may then deflect compliments and numb ourselves to positive attention because we don't feel we deserve it.

In other words, *by holding on to low body confidence and believing that your body is the only thing that makes you worthy of love, you rob yourself of the love that is all around you.*

When Heather began tapping on her own critical voice about her looks and her body, she was able to experience how body confidence was impacting her ability to enjoy herself and her relationship. As she shared in an e-mail, "Yesterday I went to the lake and wore my one-piece with NO shorts or cover-up. Feeling better about myself feels great. I think it also helps me care enough to dress better for my figure, which adds to how much better I feel. My significant other and I were much more affectionate, too!"

By using tapping to get in touch with ourselves and feel confident in our bodies, we're able to receive and give love without feeling threatened or unworthy. Heather hadn't lost any weight; she had just allowed herself to feel confident in the skin she was in. That confidence resulted in her experiencing more love.

A woman with confidence is hypnotic. A smile is mesmerizing. Presence, openness, a sense of humor—these are all things that make a woman attractive. We've all experienced the presence of someone who walks in and lights up a room. It's never about their looks but about their energy. Allow yourself to light up the room by being your beautiful self.

Now that we've explored the behaviors, events, beliefs, and emotions that may have contributed to our weight struggles up to this point, we're ready to apply a new level of awareness to how we're caring for ourselves and our bodies. In Part III, we'll look at a few important areas where we can implement lifestyle changes that increase body confidence and promote weight loss. Keep up the great work! You've already come so far.

# Feeling Confident in Your Feminine Body

**Karate Chop:** Even though it's felt unsafe to feel attractive in my body, I love and accept myself and my body. (*Repeat three times.*)

**Eyebrow:** It hasn't felt safe in my body . . .

**Side of Eye:** So I've held on to this extra weight.

**Under Eye:** It's a way to protect myself . . .

**Under Nose:** And hide.

**Chin:** But I still don't feel safe . . .

**Collarbone:** Even with this extra weight.

**Under Arm:** So I am open to a new way . . .

**Top of Head:** Of feeling safe and strong.

**Eyebrow:** I allow my body to be smaller . . .

**Side of Eye:** And my energy to be larger.

**Under Eye:** It's safe to have a smaller body.

**Under Nose:** I now feel my big energy.

**Chin:** I am safe within my big energy.

**Collarbone:** I am powerful within my big energy.

**Under Arm:** It's safe to be confident in my body.

**Top of Head:** I trust and follow my intuition.

**Eyebrow:** I am present in my body.

**Side of Eye:** I am aware of my breath.

**Under Eye:** I trust my intuition.

**Under Nose:** I have a voice.

**Chin:** I have the ability to act . . .

**Collarbone:** And I do so immediately.

**Under Arm:** What I feel matters more . . .

**Top of Head:** Than anyone else's opinion.

**Eyebrow:** Losing weight might mean I attract compliments . . .

**Side of Eye:** Or unwanted attention.

**Under Eye:** I can feel safe and strong in my body.

**Under Nose:** The more I care about what I think . . .

**Chin:** The less I care what others think.

**Collarbone:** These are just words . . .

**Under Arm:** And I have the power to react . . .

**Top of Head:** In any way that feels right to me.

**Eyebrow:** It's safe to stand in my power.

**Side of Eye:** It's safe to receive praise.

**Under Eye:** I know I am more than my body . . .

**Under Nose:** And I can still love and appreciate my body.

**Chin:** As I feel stronger emotionally, I feel stronger physically.

**Collarbone:** As I feel stronger physically, I feel stronger emotionally.

**Under Arm:** It feels good to be in my body now.

**Top of Head:** The more I take care of my body, the safer and stronger I feel.

**Eyebrow:** I feel in control . . .

**Side of Eye:** And powerful . . .

**Under Eye:** In a smaller body . . .

**Under Nose:** Within this large energy.

**Chin:** It feels freeing to be me.

**Collarbone:** I no longer need to hide.

**Under Arm:** I experience the blessing of being a woman.

**Top of Head:** I am powerful.

# Part III

# Moving Forward

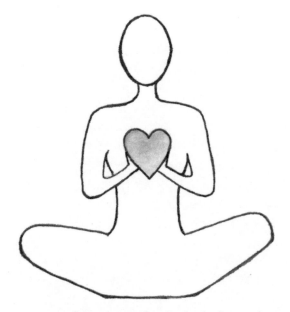

It's also helpful to realize that this body that we have,
This body that's sitting here right now . . .
and this mind that we have at this very moment,
are exactly what we need
to feel fully human, fully awake, fully alive

– Pema Chödrön

# Chapter 9

# Finding the Pleasure in Exercise

When we feel pain around body image, our relationship with exercise often falls into one of two extremes—either we avoid it or we use it as a form of self-punishment.

When we're avoiding it, exercise can seem painful because it forces us to be present in the body we have, and being present, we feel and experience our own self-neglect. *How did I let myself get like this?* we wonder. Overwhelmed by distress, we wage an internal battle with ourselves, judging our body harshly and feeling a great deal of sadness and guilt. If we are dealing with physical pain as well, the idea of exercising can bring up so much anger and frustration that the brain fires off a stress response.

If we find ourselves at the other extreme, using exercise as a form of self-punishment, we may see movement as the price we have to pay for being fat. We feel the need to torture ourselves physically the same way we torture ourselves verbally for not being "good enough." This makes exercising a habit we will never sustain because it comes from a place of pain. Once the pain lessens or something else grabs our attention, we will go back to old habits.

Many women find themselves going back and forth between these two extremes, cycling between total neglect and extreme exercise fueled by pain and panic. At both extremes, if we hate the body we have and don't show it any love and compassion, we turn exercise into something we can never enjoy. And this negative relationship with movement can throw a wrench in our weight loss and body confidence progress.

Luckily, tapping can help us create a new relationship with exercise. This is just what happened for me. No one has been as surprised as I am by how much I love the way exercise makes me feel. That's something I honestly never thought I'd be able to say!

Like me, so many of my clients have found that using tapping to create a new relationship with exercise is really a process of rediscovering what we all knew as children—that moving our body is an endless source of pleasure and enjoyment. Whatever your relationship with exercise has been up to now, if you go through this process and do the tapping, it will transform you in ways that get you up and moving for the sheer joy of it.

## Early Experiences with Exercise

"Ortner, go run three laps and when you get back, pay attention." By the end of the first lap, I was out of breath and cursing my gym teacher in my mind. With her and my soccer coach, it was the same: whenever I didn't follow directions or wasn't paying attention (which was often), I was forced to run laps. It wasn't a traumatic experience, but it did create a belief in me that running was a form of punishment.

Many of my clients also formed negative associations with exercise during their early school years when they felt out of place or that they couldn't keep up. Molly was one of those clients. Her memory of being laughed at by other girls after being hit in the head with a volleyball created a fear of exercise that stayed with her. Because of that early experience, she had a belief that exercising meant embarrassing herself. Not surprisingly, she avoided exercise.

Another client, Sharon, remembered coming in last place when she was forced to run in gym class. By the time she crossed the finish line, she was exhausted, in pain, and embarrassed as all her classmates stood there staring at her. From that day forward, she had believed that exercising was something she just wasn't good at.

Though years have passed and gym class may be a distant memory, those seemingly small events in the past can create a negative foundation for our beliefs around physical activity. If we don't address the stress the memory causes, we will continue to find reasons to avoid exercise. If just the thought of exercising causes the amygdala to fire off the fight-or-flight stress response, we'll do everything in our power to avoid exercise because it doesn't feel safe.

What is your first memory of exercise? Did some of your early memories around physical activity leave you feeling left out, embarrassed, or punished? If you discover a stressful event or discouraging memory around exercise, refer back to Chapter 5 and tap on that event until you're able to clear the stress and emotions it created.

## Exploring Beliefs Around Exercise

Whether or not they come from events in the past, often our greatest resistance to exercise lies in our beliefs. In some cases, our most limiting beliefs around exercise relate to our identity (who we are); in others, they focus on what we think is possible (what we can do). To continue unpacking the layers of our relationship with exercise so it doesn't stop us in our tracks, let's explore some of the most common negative beliefs we have in each of these areas.

### WHEN EXERCISING JUST ISN'T WHO YOU ARE

"I feel like I'm never going to lose weight because I'm not one of 'those people,'" Lucy shared one day while taking my online class. After trying to exercise at home with a workout video, she had ended up in a puddle of tears, so sure she could never be like the woman in the video. "Every time I try to exercise, I think about the athletes in school and how I could never fit in," she said.

Because exercise had been a source of emotional pain for her, Lucy had created a belief that exercise wasn't part of who she was; that she would never be "one of those people" who exercises. After Lucy and I did some tapping on her feelings of not fitting in with the athletes at school, I asked her to imagine working out—to really put herself there in her mind—and then notice what she was thinking.

"I thought of this woman I know," she said. "She's someone I really admire. She decided to participate in a walk-a-thon to bring awareness to a charity she was passionate about supporting. So she started to walk. She was seventy-two or seventy-three, and she built herself to the point where she could walk about thirty miles. That summer she participated in the walk-a-thon. It was a hundred degrees that day. She had never done anything like that before and she did it."

Why was this simple thought such a major breakthrough for Lucy? The thoughts we think when we exercise determine whether it's a pleasurable experience or not. Lucy went from avoiding exercise because it reminded her of not fitting in to associating exercise with someone inspirational she wanted to emulate. With this positive association in her mind, Lucy could begin to feel excited about exercising.

Is there someone in your life with a healthy and empowering relationship to exercise? It doesn't need to be someone you know personally. Just identifying with them or being inspired by their achievements can help you rebuild an empowering relationship with exercise.

When exercise seems outside of our identity, when we believe it's something *other* people do, we often adopt additional beliefs to support that one.

**I'm just not good at it.** Since exercise is often linked to sports in school, we sometimes think of it as a competition that we're not "good enough" to participate in. As we have seen, beliefs often shape experience. When we believe something like *I'm just not good at exercise*, that belief becomes a fixed reality, something we don't think we have the power to change.

When we get rid of that belief, we see that there is no good or bad, no winner or loser in exercise. Exercise is part of a sacred relationship we all have with our own bodies. Movement is a way to express our gratitude for being alive. We don't need to be perfect when we exercise, and we don't need to be fast or strong. We just need to support our health by moving our bodies on a regular basis.

My godmother is a great example of this. At 56 she's an avid runner, and she's in incredible shape. She runs in the early morning and loves how it feels to be outside as the sun comes up. She has no idea how far or how fast she runs. For her, running is a way to de-stress and feel powerful in her body.

Once I did tapping to clear my old beliefs that running was punishment and that running was something I could never do (every lap I'd ever run had *felt* like torture), one November I began to go for runs along the Hudson River. Inspired by my godmother's approach, I didn't time myself or have a distance in mind. I didn't try to run fast, and sometimes I walked. I just began moving with the intention of enjoying myself. What I discovered in the process was a whole new world, a new way of relating to my body. I discovered that I love how refreshing cold air feels on my skin, how inspired I feel being near the water, and how being closer to nature makes everything in my life seem more beautiful. Because I was able to clear the judgmental voice in my head, running took on a whole new meaning in my life. It has since become one of my favorite activities. I don't need to judge whether I'm good or bad at it; I just enjoy the time I spend being outside and feeling inspired.

> Lazy doesn't exist. Lazy is a symptom of something else . . . it's usually a pervasive lack of self-worth, or a feeling of helplessness. That's why fitness is so important. You have the ability to show somebody what she's capable of very quickly.
>
> —JILLIAN MICHAELS

**I don't like exercise.** When someone tells me they don't like exercise, I tell them that their body loves to exercise. What doesn't like exercise is a mind that judges and punishes itself during the process.

The fact is that the body needs movement to thrive. Research has shown that living a sedentary life is dangerous to our health and well-being. When we don't move, we have more aches and pains and increase our chances of experiencing illness and disease.

Although it's good to know the physical reasons for movement, we still won't do it if it causes us emotional pain. That's why it's so important to use tapping to create a new relationship with movement. Until we're able to create a positive emotional foundation for exercise, we simply won't.

What's the real reason you "don't like" movement? Does it cause you to feel anxiety, fear, or some other negative emotion? If you're unsure, start tapping on it. Beginning with the karate chop point, you might just say, "Even though I don't like exercise, I love and accept myself." Repeat that three times, and then keep tapping through all the points and see what you discover. And trust me: everyone can find something they enjoy doing. It may not be your standard running or jogging—these are definitely not for everyone. But there are myriad other options such as yoga, dance, walking, hiking; you just have to find the one that's right for you.

**I'm too embarrassed to work out or move my body.** It had been three years since Autumn had done any exercise. "I used to love yoga, and my friend has been encouraging me to go to a class with her, but I keep needing to reschedule. I just don't have time." She believed that her schedule wasn't allowing her to go to yoga class but I knew there had to be another reason.

"I want you to imagine walking into that yoga class. What doesn't feel safe or comfortable about that image?" I asked.

"I'm scared of so many things," she replied. At over 225 pounds Autumn felt too ashamed of her body to exercise. "I'm scared I'll start sweating heavily, that I'll be breathing heavily, that I won't be able to do a pose and people will be looking at me and judging me," she explained.

When I asked about past events that may have created this belief, she immediately said there were none; these thoughts were only in her head. Next I asked what she thought about when she exercised. "Do you judge yourself in your own mind?" I asked. She didn't hesitate before saying yes.

So often, the judgment we fear from others is actually judgment we are putting on ourselves. As we saw in Chapter 6, we often have beliefs about ourselves that are incredibly cruel and can cause us to judge ourselves harshly. As Autumn and I tapped on her fears around exercise, saying each one out loud while stimulating the tapping points, she began to relax. When we ended with a deep breath, I asked her again to imagine herself at yoga class. "I feel like everyone will be cheering me on," she said. "If I can go to yoga, anyone can. I'm actually an inspiration."

What I love about tapping is that when we clear our fear, the mind naturally finds an empowering belief or idea to replace it with. That's what happened to Autumn.

When Autumn's fear of other people's judgments was gone, her anxiety went from an intensity level of 7 down to 2. I then asked her what feelings remained. "It's more nerves around trying something new, but I'm willing to go for it. I actually can't wait." Right after our session she reached out to her friend and soon after, for the first time in three years, Autumn walked into a yoga class.

During our coaching session the following week, I asked Autumn about her yoga experience. The class had turned out to be hot yoga, so the room was intentionally set at around 100°F. The second Autumn walked in, she began to sweat, and not long after class started she realized that she couldn't do all the moves. What's fascinating is that even though all of her old fears had come true, she'd had a great time and felt proud of herself for going. Because she had cleared her self-judgment, she could see that everyone in the room was just doing their best and no one was judging her.

Since that day, Autumn has begun a weekly yoga practice and walks for 20 minutes every day. She feels more confident and comfortable in her own body than she ever has. She's having a great time moving her body and no longer feels intimidated by exercise. Instead she sees it as a chance to appreciate her body, relax her mind, and enjoy the entire experience.

## HOW IS YOUR INTERNAL DIALOGUE IMPACTING YOU?

Like Autumn, many of my clients who resist exercise realize while tapping that they have become the victim of their own internal dialogue. As we've seen, when we think negative and critical thoughts while we exercise, we prevent ourselves from experiencing the pleasure of exercise.

Do you hear a nasty judgmental voice when you move your body? Imagine the last time you worked out or did some form of physical exercise. When you have that image in your mind, what are you thinking about? Do you hear a voice that says something like:

- You're doing it wrong!

- You can't even keep up.

- You look ridiculous.

- You're too fat.

- You're too weak.

- This is torture.

- There is no point.

- You aren't "one of those people."

- Just quit.

- You're embarrassing yourself.

- Everyone's staring at you.

- How did you let yourself get like this?

So many intelligent, kind, and loving women are walking around listening to their harsh and unforgiving internal voice telling them who they are—and who they're not. When we use tapping, we can finally quiet that negative voice and give ourselves the love we've been showering on others for years.

Write down or circle the statement that best relates to you. Is there a particular emotion you feel when you think or say that statement? How true does that statement feel? Rate your answers by emotional intensity on a scale of 0 to 10. Simply giving a voice to your own fears can be incredibly effective. Here is a tapping script to help you do that:

**Karate Chop:** Even though I've been judging myself when I exercise, I love and accept myself. (*Repeat three times.*)

**Eyebrow:** This negative voice when I move my body . . .

**Side of Eye:** It points out everything I'm doing wrong.

**Under Eye:** It points out this discomfort.

**Under Nose:** It's hard to enjoy this process . . .

**Chin:** When I'm trapped within the negative thoughts in my mind.

**Collarbone:** I give these thoughts a voice now and let them go.

**Under Arm:** "You're doing it wrong."

**Top of Head:** "You can't even keep up."

**Eyebrow:** "There is no point."

**Side of Eye:** "Just quit."

**Under Eye:** "Just end this misery."

**Under Nose:** "It's too hard."

**Chin:** "You're just not good enough."

**Collarbone:** "You're embarrassing yourself."

**Under Arm:** "People are judging you."

**Top of Head:** All these voices in my head . . .

*When the intensity of your initial tapping target is 5 or lower, you can move on to the positive.*

**Eyebrow:** I hear these voices . . .

**Side of Eye:** But I can choose to believe these voices or not.

**Under Eye:** These voices begin to sound silly.

**Under Nose:** I am in control.

**Chin:** I choose to listen to the one quiet voice . . .

**Collarbone:** That says "I can do this."

**Under Arm:** I *am* doing this.

**Top of Head:** I honor myself for showing up.

**Eyebrow:** Releasing the need to be perfect . . .

**Side of Eye:** I allow my body to move.

**Under Eye:** I find peace within any discomfort.

**Under Nose:** I am doing the best I can and that is enough.

**Chin:** I am so proud of myself.

**Collarbone:** I cheer myself on.

**Under Arm:** With every step I take, I honor myself.

**Top of Head:** I may not be perfect but I am unstoppable!

*Take a deep breath and check in with how you feel. Measure the intensity again and continue tapping until you experience relief.*

# WHEN EXERCISE DOESN'T FIT INTO YOUR LIFE

When we're unconsciously resisting exercise, the other types of beliefs we often adopt are about why exercise doesn't fit into our lives. Instead of facing our internal reality (our beliefs and emotions around exercise and our bodies), we look to our external circumstances to explain why we don't (and can't) exercise. Although these beliefs are convincing at first, once we've used tapping to clear internal resistance to exercise, we find that our external circumstances easily adapt to our new desire to spend time moving our bodies. So let's look at some of these common excuses.

**I don't have time.** As we saw earlier, before she did tapping on the deeper causes of her resistance to exercise, Autumn sincerely believed she didn't have time for yoga class. Each time she said that, she offered long, complicated stories about the details of her schedule. She felt that those stories were proof that she didn't have time for exercise. When we got to the root of what was stopping her from exercising, though, we found that fear and self-judgment were the real reasons she couldn't find time for yoga class.

When we say we don't have time to exercise, we are actually saying we don't know how to face our internal reality. We don't know what to do with the emotions, stress, and maybe also the memories that are fueling our tortured relationship with exercise. That's where tapping becomes such a useful tool because it allows us to work through all of that far quicker and more easily than ever before.

We need to dig deeper and see what's underneath our "I don't have time" excuse. Take a moment now to ask yourself, *Why don't I find the time to exercise?* When you imagine yourself exercising, do you feel guilty for taking time for yourself? Do other negative feelings, voices, or memories come up? If so, what are they?

There are 1,440 minutes in a day, and all of us can use 30 of them to exercise. Some of the most successful (and busiest!) people in the world make time for exercise because they believe it's essential to their success. What is blocking you?

## How Exercise Makes You More Productive

Is it even possible to be too busy to exercise? Richard Branson, founder of Virgin Group, has started more than 400 companies. He has also published multiple books, is an active philanthropist, and has many personal hobbies. When asked how he does it all, he always lists exercise as his number-one productivity secret.

Research suggests that he may be right. Studies show that exercise increases creativity, helps you sleep better, and gives you energy, all of which make you more productive. That means that being busy is a reason to exercise more often, not less.

**I'm too tired to exercise.** We don't exercise because we're too tired, and we're too tired because we don't exercise. How can we break this nasty little cycle?

When we feel too tired to exercise, the idea that exercise will give us energy seems ridiculous. Sitting on the couch makes so much more sense! Although we may know and even believe that exercise increases energy, sometimes it's difficult to overcome fatigue on our own. Sheer willpower works occasionally, but forcing ourselves to move only reinforces the idea that exercise is punishment. Instead, we can use tapping to increase our energy first, before we begin exercising. Often, stress is the source of our fatigue. Once we lower our stress, we find that we have more energy than we realized. (Trust me: it works! I still use tapping on days when I'm not feeling up to exercising and it's just enough to get me out the door.)

Here is a simple tapping script you can use to overcome fatigue when you feel too tired to exercise:

**Karate Chop:** Even though I feel too tired to exercise, I accept how I feel. (*Repeat three times.*)

**Eyebrow:** I don't want to exercise.

**Side of Eye:** I'm exhausted . . .

**Under Eye:** And I have other things I need to do.

**Under Nose:** I'm just too exhausted.

**Chin:** All this resistance around exercising . . .

**Collarbone:** All this fatigue . . .

**Under Arm:** I just want to relax.

**Top of Head:** I just want a break.

**Eyebrow:** Maybe this can be easier than I thought.

**Side of Eye:** Maybe moving my body can be the break I need.

**Under Eye:** I'm open to making this easy.

**Under Nose:** I'm open to making this fun.

**Chin:** All I need to do is start.

**Collarbone:** I soon experience the relief . . .

**Under Arm:** And the energy I need.

**Top of Head:** I am ready to go.

## Research: Exercise Increases Energy

Research has repeatedly shown that physical activity increases energy. One study at the University of Georgia found that sedentary but otherwise healthy adults who did 20 minutes of low to moderate aerobic exercise three times a week for six consecutive weeks felt more energized and experienced less fatigue.

**Pain and/or illness prevents me from exercising.** "I abandoned myself. Overnight I stopped doing all the things that make me happy," Marci shared. Diagnosed with the autoimmune disease Hashimoto's in 2007, she experienced such extreme fatigue that she stopped doing the biking, dancing, and yoga she had always loved. As the months turned into years, she gradually gained 50 pounds, which felt like double that on her small frame. Feeling heavy and ugly, she began telling herself that if she couldn't do all of the yoga poses she once had, and if she couldn't climb all of the hills in her neighborhood on her bike, there was no point in exercising.

After tapping on her stress, as well as her anger and frustration with her body, Marci experienced a huge shift. After years of feeling like she couldn't exercise, she began to bike again and do daily yoga poses. Instead of seeing exercise as a competition with her physically fit, pre-illness self, she began to approach it as something that makes her feel good. No longer beating herself up for not being able to bike up the longest and steepest hills, she simply got off her bike and walked it to the top. Whether she was on her bike or walking next to it, being outside moving her body made her feel good. It was the first time since her diagnosis that Marci had been able to see herself as a woman who *has* a disease, rather than a woman who is her disease.

When we're dealing with health issues, we often face very real limitations around what the body can do. While we may not be able to do everything, through tapping we often see that it's the stress and emotions around our health issues that are preventing us from exercising. Once we're able to accept our limitations and use tapping to clear the stress, emotions, and physical pain that our health condition(s) has created, we see that we actually can do some kinds of exercise. (There are even workout videos you can do while sitting in a chair.)

When we are loving and patient with ourselves, we can create a new relationship with the body and the illness and/or pain that has been limiting us. Most important, we find that exercise makes us feel better, not just physically but also emotionally. Numerous studies have demonstrated the mental, emotional, and physical benefits of exercise, which include preventing diabetes and heart disease, increasing flexibility and energy, improving sleep, and relieving and preventing anxiety and depression. With tapping, physical limitations don't need to prevent us from moving the body. Instead, our health issues become our greatest inspiration for exercising.

## The Myth of an End Goal

Before I began using tapping to address my weight issues, I had always looked at exercise as a means to an end goal—weight loss. Every time I got on an "exercising kick," I would get passionate about a new video or class at the gym, mark my weight on the calendar, and begin a food journal. As days and weeks passed, though, my fuel would run low. Before long I would stop exercising altogether.

Because exercise was what I thought people did to lose weight, when I saw physically fit women at the gym I'd think, *Why are you still here?* As far as I was concerned, they already looked great, so they no longer needed to punish themselves with exercise. Not surprisingly, every time I lost the weight, I would stop exercising and regain it.

After several years of this same pattern repeating itself, I realized that "to lose weight" wasn't an empowering enough reason for me to exercise consistently. I began to question everything I thought about exercise and became curious about why some people successfully make exercise part of their daily lives.

The journey I've been on since has completely transformed my life. By changing how I relate to exercise and allowing myself to love it—not just the running I mentioned, but all different kinds of exercise—I have stepped into a new world where I feel strong and confident, energetic and beautiful. Although I still have days when I feel too tired or busy to exercise, moving my body has become such an important part of my life that I literally can't imagine not exercising on a regular basis.

## Why Exercise: Emotional and Physical Benefits

I have always believed in turning jealousy into curiosity, so for a time, whenever I saw someone on the street who was physically fit, I asked them what motivated them to exercise consistently. (Yes, I actually stopped strangers to interview them—I still do, about all kinds of topics.) After receiving answers from dozens of people, I couldn't help but notice that none of them ever said "to burn calories" or "to lose weight." Their first response was almost always about the emotional benefits they got from exercise. Physical benefits came second. Over and over again, people said things like, "Exercise helps me de-stress," "It's my time for myself," or "I always feel better after I exercise."

Over time, these consistent responses made me realize that I had never really given exercise a chance. I was too busy judging myself to experience the emotional benefits that come from moving my body. I began to wonder . . . what if, like tapping, moving my body was a healing modality in itself? If I saw exercise as a spiritual experience, would moving my body feel different?

By that point in my journey, I was clear on the beliefs and patterns that had caused me to hold on to the weight. I was rebellious, courageous, and determined, but I also often suppressed my true self to please others. The bottom line was that I was scared to take up space in this world, so I played small in a large body that I hoped would protect me from the pain I was already feeling.

Once I began to tap on my resistance to exercise and could look at it in a new way, I realized that exercise was essential to my healing journey. Soon

> To sweat is to pray, to make an offering of your innermost self. Sweat is holy water, prayer beads, pearls of liquid that release your past. . . . Sweat is an ancient and universal form of self healing.
>
> —GABRIELLE ROTH

after, I took a kickboxing class that turned that belief into a very personal reality. During that class, for the first time ever, I experienced in my body what it feels like to discover my own power and voice. I realized that I could push energy out of my body instead of always absorbing other people's energy. It was a huge turning point for me, and I left that class feeling more powerful than I had in years.

Kickboxing soon became a way for me to process anger, an emotion I had been too ashamed to feel. Yoga has since taught me how to listen to my body and "go with the flow." I often leave a class feeling that it was even better for my soul than my body.

It's important to realize that we cannot experience our own true power and essence if we don't move. Movement, like tapping, helps us

## The Top Ten Reasons I Exercise

Now that I'm like the people I used to stop on the street to interview about why they exercise, I thought I'd share why I now make a point of moving my body:

1. As my friend Erin Stutland says, "Movement in your body means movement in your life." Over and over again, I've seen how true that is for me and my life. When I'm feeling stuck, I know I need to move.
2. Movement is an expression of gratitude toward my body for all it does for me.
3. Movement makes me feel connected to my body and its intelligence, which helps me make better decisions and keeps me feeling like my best self.
4. I'm smarter and more creative when I'm exercising. (Research backs this up; exercise causes increased blood flow to the brain, which stimulates the creative centers in the brain.)

process emotions. Once we use tapping to peel back and release limiting beliefs about exercise, we can receive an even deeper form of healing through exercise itself. Exercise isn't about achieving an end goal; it's about having a present-moment experience that connects us with ourselves, our body, and our own power.

## Practical Tips for Beginning to Exercise

After tapping through your resistance to exercise—the stress, emotional blocks, physical pain, and anything else that may be affecting

5. Movement is a spiritual experience for me, like a physical form of prayer or a moving meditation.
6. Movement makes me feel strong, confident, beautiful, and sexy, like a force to be reckoned with.
7. Movement helps me be in the present moment, which helps me feel at peace.
8. Movement is one of the ways I show myself love, so when I exercise, I'm reminding myself that I'm worthy of my own love.
9. Movement makes me feel playful and energetic.
10. Movement makes me feel powerful in a deep and authentic way.

Notice what's missing here? "Burning calories" and "losing weight" appear exactly nowhere on my list.

Why will you choose to exercise? Do you want to feel more energetic and playful with your children? Do you want to experience more creativity and productivity in your life? What might inspire you to get up and get moving? Feel free to write down your own Top Reasons Why I Exercise list, and keep adding to it as you discover new ones.

how you think and feel about exercise—you may surprise yourself by feeling slightly excited about the idea of moving your body. To help you take advantage of that momentum, here are some practical tips that my clients and I have found helpful over the years.

**Make exercise non-negotiable.** A friend once said to me, "People don't struggle with exercise. They struggle with making the decision to exercise." Often, we spend so much time thinking that we "should" exercise that it starts to feel like this incredibly overwhelming decision. If we stopped thinking about it and just went ahead and did it, we'd be done exercising before we knew it, and more important, we'd feel great! That's why Nike's "Just do it" slogan strikes a chord with so many people. When we stop overthinking exercise and make it non-negotiable, we get to experience how great it makes us feel.

**Find an exercise buddy and/or some support.** Research has shown that people who work out with some kind of support group get better results. When you look for support, I encourage you to find someone who is in better shape than you. Sometimes when two people at the same fitness level try to support each other, they end up falling back into old patterns, finding comfort in the fact that they are falling together. The better bet is to find someone who's been exercising regularly for a long time, someone who's excited about you loving exercise as much as they do.

Why would someone who exercises consistently want to be your buddy? Even the most committed fitness enthusiasts have busy lives that occasionally interfere with their desire to stay consistent. They may really appreciate your support. It's also fun! My friend Sarah is my fitness buddy. She has always used her family history of heart disease as motivation to stay in shape. She says she feels most like herself when she's on her bike. We don't work out together, but we do text each other most mornings with motivation that gets us up and going. Sometimes we set fun fitness challenges for ourselves. Other times, we encourage each other to get out in spite of bad weather. The reality is that there are some days (especially in the dark and cold of winter) when it takes a little more energy to get up and go. Having a fitness buddy makes that easier and more fun.

**Make exercise fun.** When Autumn started going to yoga for the first time in three years, she let herself try different yoga classes until she found one she loved. Give yourself permission to experiment with how you can make movement more fun. Try a dance class, order a fun fitness DVD, or go for a walk in a local park. You can mix and match different exercise options depending on your mood on a given day.

Some days, adding in an enjoyable distraction may be what you need. When I texted my friend Natalie asking her how she gets herself motivated to exercise when she doesn't feel like it, she replied with two words: *True Blood.* How does a show about vampires help her work out? She downloaded the episodes on her phone and only allows herself to watch them while she's on the treadmill. This makes her workout fun and easy. "I get so into the show that before I know it, it's over and I've been on the treadmill for an hour. I got to watch my favorite show and I feel great."

> Food is the most widely abused antianxiety drug in America, and exercise is the most potent yet underutilized antidepressant.
>
> —BILL PHILLIPS

I love to work out on the elliptical while reading historical fiction. I get so involved in the story that I don't even want to get off. (If you own a Kindle or other reading device, you can make the text bigger, which makes it a lot easier to read when you're moving.)

And then there's always my personal favorite . . . If walls could talk, my solo dance parties would be the talk of the town! From jumping off couches to attempting the moonwalk with my socks on a wooden floor, I love to dance by myself! I do not hold back. Sometimes I'm Shakira, and other times I'm Tina Turner. Whatever the case, I'm always having fun. If you haven't done any physical activity for a while, begin by just dancing in your living room. Find your favorite song and let the music move you. Start discovering how silly and playful you can be when you move. Let's stop making movement a serious burden; instead, let's make it an expression of joy and gratitude for being alive.

Whatever kind of exercise you're doing on any given day, make a point of asking yourself how you can make it even more pleasurable, whether that means watching your favorite show while exercising at a gym, dancing wildly, or working out outdoors so you can look at beautiful flowers.

**Let yourself find comfort in discomfort.** I've always noticed that the first ten minutes of exercising is when I'm most tempted to quit. It's when everything hurts and I feel short of breath. If I keep exercising, it gets easier. After years of noticing this, I finally did some research and learned that those first ten minutes feel harder for everyone, including elite athletes. It's when your body is adjusting to exercise. The difficulty you feel is the lag time that happens as your body begins delivering adequate fuel to your muscles.

Keep this in mind when you start exercising, and don't take that initial discomfort as a sign that you can't do it. Instead of stopping, try focusing on positive thoughts that keep you going. With practice you'll find that it's easier to get comfortable with that short stretch of discomfort at the start.

**Use affirmations when you move.** A woman in my program shared that she chanted, "I may be slow, but I go even when I could say no." Saying this mantra over and over again helped her lose 110 pounds!

When I run and feel myself struggling during those first ten minutes, I say to myself, "Steady and smooth." I don't need to force the movement or go at top speed; I just find ways to make my running "smoother." Because that sounds easy and effortless, it motivates me to keep going.

Erin Stutland's workouts are another favorite of mine because they combine movement with positive affirmations. After becoming a fan of her work, I later had the honor of becoming close friends with her. Her approach to exercise makes movement an empowering and fun experience. If you haven't yet tried the fun workout she and I created together, I encourage you to watch it at www.TheTappingSolution .com/chapter9.

At the end of the workout, we do some of the dance moves I've mastered through my solo dance parties. If seeing me look ridiculous helps relieve your fear of looking ridiculous when you exercise, I am happy to oblige!

**Never underestimate the power of a walk.** Plato, Aristotle, Albert Einstein, and Steve Jobs—some of the most brilliant minds in our history were avid walkers. Walking is a great way to exercise, overcome fatigue, decrease stress, and increase brain function and creativity. Steve Jobs was famous for holding meetings during long walks. He even designed the new Apple campus specifically to accommodate walking meetings. In a similarly innovative spirit, one of my students began doing her tapping while taking a walk. Great idea!

# Finding the Pleasure in Exercise

**Karate Chop:** Even though I have all this resistance to exercise, I love and accept myself. *(Repeat three times.)*

**Eyebrow:** I just don't have the time.

**Side of Eye:** I don't have the energy.

**Under Eye:** I don't want to.

**Under Nose:** There are so many other things I need to do.

**Chin:** It's uncomfortable.

**Collarbone:** It feels like torture.

**Under Arm:** I feel depleted of energy . . .

**Top of Head:** The thought of exercising is exhausting.

**Eyebrow:** I logically know this will help my energy . . .

**Side of Eye:** But it doesn't feel true.

**Under Eye:** I'm getting clear on what's under this resistance.

**Under Nose:** I know I should go . . .

**Chin:** But I'm rebelling against this pressure.

**Collarbone:** Maybe I don't *have* to exercise.

**Under Arm:** Maybe I can *choose* to exercise.

**Top of Head:** All this remaining resistance . . .

**Eyebrow:** I don't want to face that critical voice . . .

**Side of Eye:** That says I'm not good enough . . .

**Under Eye:** That says to stop trying . . .

**Under Nose:** That judges every movement . . .

**Chin:** That judges my body.

**Collarbone:** I face that voice now.

**Under Arm:** As it loses its power . . .

**Top of Head:** I begin to hear a new voice.

**Eyebrow:** I am good enough.

**Side of Eye:** I can do this.

**Under Eye:** I can even enjoy this.

**Under Nose:** I don't need to be perfect.

**Chin:** I do my best.

**Collarbone:** I enjoy the moment.

**Under Arm:** As I connect with my body . . .

**Top of Head:** I connect to a greater wisdom.

**Eyebrow:** Ideas begin to flow.

**Side of Eye:** I feel strong and resourceful.

**Under Eye:** I feel clear and confident.

**Under Nose:** When I feel stuck in my life . . .

**Chin:** I begin to move my body.

**Collarbone:** When there is movement in my body . . .

**Under Arm:** There is movement in my life.

**Top of Head:** Life begins to flow.

**Eyebrow:** I begin to fall in love with the feelings that come from movement.

**Side of Eye:** I notice my own strength and power.

**Under Eye:** There is no place to arrive to . . .

**Under Nose:** I enjoy being in my body.

**Chin:** Movement is an expression of gratitude for my body.

**Collarbone:** I enjoy this time for myself.

**Under Arm:** I realize my potential through movement.

**Top of Head:** I love to move.

## Chapter 10

# Untangling the Myths, Facts, and Feelings Around Food

Food has become such a tortured topic for so many of us that it is often a stressful block in our weight loss and body confidence journey. We try and try to eat the "right" foods to lose weight, but in spite of our efforts to choose "diet" and "healthy" foods, we can never seem to lose the weight and keep it off. We then blame ourselves or wonder if there's something wrong with our bodies, when in fact, as we'll see in this chapter, much of the "diet" and "healthy" food we're being sold works against us, robbing us of the essential nutrients the body desperately needs. Using tapping, we can finally put an end to this frustrating cycle and begin sensing what foods the body needs not only to lose weight but to feel energetic and vibrant.

## Ending the Dieting Cycle

Whenever clients or students start to lose weight, I try to connect with them to learn more about their experiences. As we've seen, we have several layers of emotions and beliefs that can hold us back. I'm always interested to learn what has had the biggest impact on their journey.

I often find that before they lost weight, they changed their eating habits, but without dieting or following any "rules" of healthy eating. And often, they didn't notice the shifts in their eating until I asked about them. As we've seen throughout this book, changes in eating seem to happen almost unconsciously. After tapping through their emotions and beliefs, many of these women gravitate toward more nourishing foods, and they enjoy the way healthier foods make them feel.

Anne, a 57-year-old retiree from Ohio, shared how the changes happened for her.

> Without all the emotions in the way, I can focus on how my body really feels. I think at some level I knew what foods weren't working for me, but I ignored how I felt and just depended on what other people told me I should eat. Dieting was so stressful! When I began to connect with my body through tapping, I was able to see what works for me, and which foods were causing symptoms . . . I used to try to push through these symptoms. Now I'm more in tune with how my body feels and what works for me. I'm not afraid of food anymore. It's so freeing!

This is the magic of tapping. Once we address underlying emotions and beliefs, we can finally connect with the body and allow it to determine what foods work best for us. The body tries to get our attention through symptoms such as fatigue, bloating, gas, acid reflux, headaches, and stuffed sinuses, showing us that something below the surface isn't right. Instead of welcoming this important information, we often feel like the body is betraying us. With tapping, we can break this cycle and make changes based on the signals the body is sending.

I see wellness as a pyramid; at the base are emotions and beliefs, then up from there, movement and nutrition. If we don't work on the emotional aspects, not only do we suffer from stress hormones that work against us, but we also fall short in moving the body and eating food that supports health. The challenge is that we have become so inundated with nutritional information and fad diets that the question "What should I eat?" has become incredibly overwhelming. We often leave it up to the "experts" without realizing that our own body is the best expert of all. Or, consumed by our stress, we give up and settle for what's convenient and cheap.

# The Perfect Storm

When it comes to our relationship with weight, food, and the body, we're stuck in a perfect storm of high stress levels, contradictory diet information, and an abundance of cheap and convenient food that is harmful to our health. With tapping we have a powerful way to manage stress and get in touch with the body. What is less obvious is the truth behind the diet, nutrition, and food information we're exposed to every day through the media and other sources.

To begin exploring some of these hidden truths, let's first take a look at a couple of national health statistics: According to the Centers for Disease Control and Prevention (CDC) more than 69 percent of Americans are overweight. In 1973, 4.2 million Americans were diagnosed with diabetes. By 2010, that number had climbed to 21.1 million.

We're so used to seeing outrageous numbers like this that we rarely stop to think about them. So take a moment now and let them really sink in. That's almost a fivefold increase in diabetes *in fewer than 40 years*.

Many people explain away the problem by saying that Americans are lazy. We eat too much and we don't exercise. I don't buy it. We're a country of intelligent, hardworking people. Something else is in play. It's not just how much we are eating but also *what* we are eating.


# Why You Can't Have Just One

Most of us don't realize when we walk into a grocery store that many of the options we're looking at, particularly packaged goods, have been specifically designed to make us eat more than the body needs.

Inside the food industry, it's called the "bliss point" and billions of dollars are spent finding it. According to Michael Moss's *New York Times* best-selling book, *Salt Sugar Fat*, the bliss point was originally perfected in soda and has since been applied to other processed foods and drinks.

Much of the packaged "food" we see in our stores is made in laboratories run by high-level scientists and mathematicians who engineer ingredients like salt, sugar, and fat as well as "food formulations" to create food products that produce high profits. These "food formulations" are not recipes. There are no chefs or bakers, and very little, if any, of our packed food is created in a normal kitchen.

We need to understand that the cards have been stacked against us. We're not low on willpower. We're not pigs or slobs. Food manufacturers are investing enormous amounts of money in creating food products, including supposedly healthy foods, that overwhelm our taste buds and keep us reaching for more. By design, these food products force us to ignore the body's signals that it is full and eat something that doesn't make us feel good. They are literally engineered to make us overeat.

The bottom line is that there's nothing wrong with us, but there is a lot wrong with much of the so-called food we're sold in boxes and packages. While our emotions may initially cause us to turn to these foods for comfort, once we taste them they grab hold of us and we can't stop. Millions of dollars are also spent on producing and distributing commercials that depict thin, happy people eating these same processed foods. The ads are designed to play on our emotions, selling us on ideas that make no sense and aren't even remotely true. We hear slogans like Kit Kat's "Gimme a break" or "Hungry? Grab a Snickers" and get tricked into associating these so-called foods with positive things, when in truth they don't give us the break we need or fully satisfy our hunger.

Many of us aren't eating real food anymore; we're eating boxes of food products. As Michael Pollan, author of *In Defense of Food: An Eater's Manifesto,* writes, ". . . while it used to be that food was all you could eat, today there are thousands of other edible foodlike substances in the supermarket." Comedian Mike Birbiglia made a similar point on Twitter, although in a more humorous way, sharing, "I think maybe the key to eating healthy is not eating any food that has a TV commercial." I think he has a valid point!

# Food Manufacturers Feed Our Fears

Food manufacturers have also caught on to our cultural obsession with health and weight loss and are now covering their boxes with labels like "whole wheat," "real fruit," and "heart healthy." Unfortunately, as we've seen, many of these so-called healthy foods are also highly processed. As just one example of how deceptive food labeling can be, here's a list of cereals that are labeled as containing "heart healthy whole grains":

> If you're concerned about your health, you should probably avoid products that make health claims. Why? Because a health claim on a food product is a strong indication it's not really food, and food is what you want to eat.
>
> —MICHAEL POLLAN

- Kix
- Trix
- Count Chocula
- Cinnamon Toast Crunch
- Lucky Charms

While these cereals may contain a select few whole grains, they're also loaded with sugar and artificial ingredients that can be harmful to our health. When we stop to pay attention, we can begin to feel the way these foods impact us.

# The Low-Fat/Fat-Free Trap

Fat-free and low-fat products are often just as bad; they're also full of sugar and artificial ingredients. Usually when food manufacturers remove fat, they add extra sugar (and often salt, or sodium, as well) to enhance the flavor. Two great examples are low-fat fruit yogurt and fat-free salad dressings. Both are sugar bombs.

Eating diet foods can also trigger an unexpected response. According to Michael Moss in *Salt Sugar Fat*, when food manufacturers want to boost sales of a certain product, they create a "healthy" and/or diet version of that food, knowing that people will get tired of eating the "healthy" version and return to buying the original. That's exactly what happened when Oreos introduced its 100-calorie packs. Not long after the "diet" 100-calorie packs hit store shelves, sales of original Oreos took off.

Like so many of my students and clients, for years I lived on diet foods and other foods I thought were healthy. I ate rice cakes not because I had a craving for Styrofoam but because I thought they'd help me lose weight. When I was able to calm my stress and emotions around food by using tapping, I could clearly see that I didn't want one rice cake; I wanted the entire pack. As it turns out, rice cakes quickly raise your blood sugar, leaving you craving sweets and other "quick fix" carbohydrates. So in my attempt to eat well, I was actually feeding my cravings.

The same is true of diet soda. In spite of its "no calories" claim, diet soda has increasingly been linked to Type 2 diabetes, regardless of body weight. Because the artificial sweeteners are a lot sweeter than real sugar, they trick your body into pumping out insulin, which slows your metabolism, increases belly fat, and increases cravings for sugar and starchy foods like bread and pasta.

These days, if a food label says it is diet, fat free, or sugar free, I don't eat it. If it says gluten free or organic, I look closely at the label and ingredients list. Real food doesn't need a label to clarify that it's healthy, so if it has a label, we need to stop and see if it's real food or a processed food product. When we can see what's really in our food and use tapping to clear our emotions and stay in touch with the body, we can notice how various foods make us feel.

# Overcoming the "Never Enough" Mentality

Another challenge we often face is a mentality of lack around food. When we first met Dr. Peta Stapleton, we were looking at her study results about how tapping supports weight loss. Just as she and I were finishing our interview about her recent study findings, I spontaneously asked her one last question: "Dr. Stapleton, by any chance, in your years of working with overweight and obese patients, have you noticed any pattern in their mentality and/or behavior?"

"Yes," she responded with a quick and firm certainty. Many women who struggle with obesity, she told me, also tend to be hoarders. She found that even after they had eliminated their cravings, the women in her study didn't want to throw away the unhealthy foods they no longer wanted to eat.

Dr. Stapleton and her team realized that these women, who were generally 40 to 50 years old, had been taught never to throw away food by their mothers and grandmothers, who had grown up during the Great Depression and World Wars (I and II) when food was scarce. As a result, they felt that they needed to stuff their kitchens and pantries full of food products "just in case."

As Dr. Stapleton shared, "We're living in an interesting time. We are constantly surrounded by food in the Western world but we have a lack mentality." People feel they need to hoard food or eat it all even though we live in a world where food is incredibly abundant.

This lack mentality is also reinforced by dieting. We often overeat sweet treats because we know that tomorrow we'll start a strict diet and suffer from deprivation. When we focus on foods we're "not allowed to eat" instead of focusing on learning about healthier options, we're more likely to fall back into a diet mentality, which often comes with a little voice that says, "Eat all of this now, as fast as you can, because you won't be allowed to later." Anytime we experience emotions of lack or deprivation around food, we are more likely to resort to over-eating as a form of rebellion.

One woman in my class shared that she ate leftover pasta late at night. She reasoned that if she didn't eat it, no one would, and tossing out the pasta simply didn't feel like an option. When she tapped on this habit, she had a big Aha! moment. She had grown up hearing her mother say she needed to eat everything on her plate because there were starving children in Africa. By eating the pasta, however, she wasn't showing gratitude for the food or solving world hunger; she was simply hurting her body by consuming more food than it could handle.

Let's do some tapping on the inability to throw food away—even if you don't want it.

Imagine you have food in your house that isn't aligned with your health goals. If you don't have the ability to donate it to a food bank, how do you feel about tossing it out? Does it create any anxiety? What thoughts come to mind? Do you believe throwing it away is "wasting money" so you'd rather eat it even if it's harmful to your body? Take some time to reflect on any emotions or thoughts around letting go of food that doesn't serve you. Measure your emotions or belief on a scale of 0 to 10 and begin to tap. This tapping script may help.

> **Karate Chop:** Even though I have to eat all of this so it doesn't go to waste, I accept how I feel and I choose to see this another way. (*Repeat three times.*)
>
> **Eyebrow:** I have to finish this.
>
> **Side of Eye:** It would be wasteful if I didn't.
>
> **Under Eye:** I'd seem ungrateful if I didn't.
>
> **Under Nose:** I need to hold on to all this food and eat it.
>
> **Chin:** This fear of letting go . . .
>
> **Collarbone:** This fear of being wasteful . . .
>
> **Under Arm:** These beliefs I picked up from my parents . . .

**Top of Head:** I'm open to seeing this another way.

**Eyebrow:** It's okay to not finish what's on my plate.

**Side of Eye:** I'm not a child who will be scolded.

**Under Eye:** I am a woman looking out for my well-being.

**Under Nose:** In order to do what I thought was morally right . . .

**Chin:** I've put my body under a lot of strain.

**Collarbone:** Eating this food won't make someone else less hungry.

**Under Arm:** I find other ways to show gratitude and help someone less fortunate.

**Top of Head:** I can throw out food that doesn't serve my body.


## The Dangers of the "Buying in Bulk" Culture

In a world where food is abundant and we are surrounded by so-called food bargains, many of us find ourselves stockpiling packaged food that is neither healthy nor nourishing. As we've seen, the same "food" that we can purchase in bulk and on sale is also engineered to make us overeat. But because many of us have been taught to hoard, when we find a sale, instead of buying one or two boxes of cereal, for example, we find ourselves buying six or eight or ten.

This mentality tends to flare up during times of financial struggle, when money seems scarce. Food marketers are aware of this and respond accordingly, knowing that when we see a sale for diet soda, we will buy it in bulk. While our conscious intention is positive—to save money—when we go for these deals, we are overlooking a critical question: *What does the body really need and want to feel great and be healthy?*

In his book *Mindless Eating: Why We Eat More Than We Think*, Brian Wansink, Ph.D., shares what he calls "The Curse of the Warehouse Club." After conducting a two-week study of bulk food buyers, he found that people ate far higher quantities of bulk food "bargains" in the first week after buying them. After that, most people lost the desire for these foods. Some then forced themselves to overeat what was left to make room for new foods, while others simply threw away what was left.

For both groups, buying in bulk caused people to overeat "foods" that don't nourish their bodies and weren't even satisfying. As we've seen, these "foods" are engineered to make us overindulge, but because they're convenient, cheap, and available everywhere at a "bargain" price, we gravitate toward them. What's worse, we may even spend more money on so-called bargains than we would if we bought just the quantity of wholesome, nourishing foods the body actually needs.

## What's in Your Grocery Bag?

One day as I was unpacking my groceries, I couldn't help but notice how pretty my bag looked. Overflowing with fresh fruits and veggies, I was struck by how bright and beautiful it was. I proudly texted a picture of my bag to Brenna, my sister-in-law and best friend since seventh grade. She is also a holistic health coach.

After seeing the photo, she called me to share a childhood memory. She remembered as a young girl seeing grocery bags in cartoons and coloring books full of colorful fruits and veggies. She wondered why the grocery bags she saw people holding as they walked out of stores now never looked like that. Instead of being full of colorful produce, they were full of boxes.

Notice your grocery bag. Is it full of fresh food or lots of boxes?

Many of us who struggle with weight fall into that "force ourselves to overeat what's left to make room for new food" category. Often it's not even a conscious decision. We may even feel buyer's remorse after purchasing something that isn't aligned with our goals. Because we still have a lack mentality, however, throwing food out doesn't feel like an option. Instead, we force ourselves to eat it and think, *I'll start a diet tomorrow.*

I used to have this exact same hoarding mentality. Every time I wanted to start a new diet, I first ate everything in my kitchen that was bad for me. This was not a leisurely, graceful meal—more like stuffing it all down my throat in a single standing. After all, I didn't want to "waste it."

The reality is that we can't hoard freshly picked apples. When we're talking about highly processed "food"—bars, chips, cookies, and premade meals—we need to face the facts. Eating these things won't solve world hunger. The bottom line is that calling Doritos (and all highly processed edible products) "food" is questionable. It's time to take a closer look at what we're putting in our mouths.

## What Is Your Body Trying to Tell You?

Even when we think we're following all the "rules" of healthy eating, when we tune in to the body, we often realize that we've been ignoring the signals it has been sending us. When we look to the body as our guide, we see that the "rules" of what works and what doesn't change from one person to the next. Relying heavily on advice and information from outside experts just doesn't work.

The reality is that our food landscape has drastically changed and we haven't been able to stop and consciously become aware of how these foods are impacting us. In fact, more and more people are experiencing adverse reactions to very common foods. A 2008 study published by the CDC found that between 1997 and 2007 there had been a 17 percent increase in food allergies in young people (under age 18).

Some areas of the country have also seen a dramatic rise in hospital visits as a result of food allergies. While the reasons for these statistics are unclear, they do suggest that we each need to pay closer attention to how our own body reacts to different foods.

## Food Allergies and Sensitivities

Sometimes, the foods we crave most—the ones we feel like we can't live without and can't stop eating after we take that first bite—are the ones we're most allergic or sensitive to. That was the case for me with baked goods. Whether it was a box of crackers I had to eat in a single sitting or an enormous plate of cookies, my cravings were incredibly intense. Even after using tapping to overcome the emotional issues behind my cravings, I found that it was best for me not to stock these items in my house. As we've seen, many of these foods are designed to make it difficult to have only one.

> Let food be thy medicine and medicine be thy food.
>
> — HIPPOCRATES

When I eliminated wheat, what was left of my cravings vanished. I also lost an enormous amount of bloat, including in my face. I suddenly had much more energy, no longer struggled with constipation, and no longer had a runny nose each morning. I was amazed that one dietary change had made that much difference.

My brother Alex had a very similar experience with dairy. Nearly all of my childhood memories include scenes of Alex blowing his nose. Literally, for years on end, his nose was either running or attached to a tissue. My mom took him from doctor to doctor, who all kept prescribing allergy medicine. By high school, Claritin was a daily part of his life.

Years later Alex tried cutting out cheese. He wasn't happy about it—cheese was his favorite food in the world! When he tried it, though, his body felt so good that there was no turning back. He no longer spent the first 30 minutes in the morning blowing his nose. He was amazed by how much better he felt.

## Using Real Food to Heal the Body

If you're interested in learning more about using the power of food to transform health and wellness, I highly recommend Dr. Mark Hyman's work. He has changed the lives of many thousands of people (including former President Bill Clinton!) who now wake up each morning feeling and looking great. Because he's a personal friend of my family, I can also vouch for what a great person he is and how incredibly dedicated he is to helping people enjoy true and vibrant health every single day.

You can listen to an interview I did with Dr. Hyman here: www .TheTappingSolution.com/chapter10.

Alex had a very obvious and fairly fast shift, which isn't always the case. What's interesting is that when Alex visits our family in Argentina, he can eat his favorite indulgence—grilled provolone cheese—without any reaction. That may be because it's hand-crafted local cheese, not processed cheese.

For Alex and many others, it's not just what we're eating but the quality of what we're eating that matters. The more processed a food is, the more likely it is that the body will have adverse reactions to it. The key for Alex was being able to notice how his body reacted to certain foods and adjust his diet accordingly.

Make the intention to eat slowly and notice how your body feels after a meal. Excess weight, bloating, gas, constipation, diarrhea, stuffy nose, low energy, and frequent headaches can all be signs that you're having an adverse reaction to a certain food. Become your own detective and discover how you feel when you eliminate certain foods. When you invest more time in your relationship with your body, you can see that it's not betraying you; it's simply trying to get your attention. It's time to listen.

# When Your Body Confuses You—Cravings and Detox

As we've seen, our strongest cravings can be for the foods we're allergic or sensitive to. Sometimes when we eliminate those same foods, we experience detox symptoms for several days. That happened to me when I stopped eating wheat. All of my symptoms—bloating, low energy, constipation—got worse at first. I was also incredibly emotional, got bad headaches, and felt very shaky. When I tapped on those symptoms, they diminished. Without tapping, there is no way I would have been able to complete the process. Once I did, I literally felt better than I ever had in my entire life. The differences in my mood, energy, and body were huge.

For some people, tapping prevents detox symptoms. That was the case for Ellie, whose body responded immediately when she was finally able to end her Diet Sunkist addiction by tapping. In addition to feeling less bloated and having less gas, she was amazed by how easy the process was with tapping. Before, she explained, "I was seriously powerless when it came to a can of Diet Sunkist. Now, nothing . . . I have gone through some serious stuff and thought that I would have to have a Diet Sunkist to feel better. I had one. Nothing. No thrill, no calm, just nothing. It wasn't even tasty. I didn't finish it. For real and true, it is in my past and out of my body!"

If you decide to try eliminating various foods to see how your body reacts, make sure to use tapping, and don't let standard detox symptoms deter you. They're a normal and healthy sign that your body is getting rid of substances that interfere with your health.

# Your Body Is Hungry for Nutrition

Now that we've looked at the ways processed food products may be negatively affecting health, the question remains—what *should* we eat?

The ultimate answer to that question is one only you can provide. Once you've tapped through your limiting emotions and beliefs, you'll be able to get in touch with your body and your intuition. When that happens, your body will usually tell you what it needs. So many of my students and clients find themselves effortlessly gravitating toward fresh fruits and veggies and away from processed foods.

Let's do some tapping now around getting in touch with our bodies and learning to trust them to guide us:

**Karate Chop:** Even though I don't know what to eat, I choose to feel calm and trust my intuition. (*Repeat three times.*)

**Eyebrow:** As I quiet my mind . . .

**Side of Eye:** And feel centered in my body . . .

**Under Eye:** I begin to notice the extra love and nourishment my body needs.

**Under Nose:** I trust my intuition as it leads me to healthy choices.

**Chin:** I become curious about how to support my body.

**Collarbone:** This is fun and easy.

**Under Arm:** I take it one choice at a time.

**Top of Head:** I'm attracted to foods that help my body thrive.

**Eyebrow:** I bring new awareness to how my body feels.

**Side of Eye:** What I thought was my body betraying me . . .

**Under Eye:** Is my body trying to get my attention.

**Under Nose:** I become curious as to how I react to foods.

**Chin:** I begin to experiment to find what's right for me.

**Collarbone:** I let go of needing to know the answer now.

**Under Arm:** I am open, curious, and patient . . .

**Top of Head:** As I become aware of how my body reacts to certain foods.

While the body often knows best, it's also important to understand that the body needs nourishment and nutrition. Food products that contain ingredients that are unfamiliar and/or unpronounceable probably aren't real food. And food products with very long ingredients lists require a closer look.

Again, the labeling of food products is incredibly misleading. As one example, the Nutri-Grain yogurt bars label reads, "More of the whole grains your body needs" and "Excellent source of calcium." Even its name, "Nutri-," suggests that the contents are nutritious. When you look at the label, though, these bars contain 56 ingredients. Why is that? Personally, I've never cooked anything that needs 56 ingredients. Also, I'm no diet expert but I do know that "Red 40" doesn't grow on a tree, and most of the other ingredients are impossible to pronounce. Common sense tells me this is not ideal for my body even though other things on the label tell me otherwise.

When we consume products like these, the body can become deprived of the actual nutrients and nutrition it needs. In his book *The Gabriel Method*, Jon Gabriel explains how this lack of nutrition impacts weight. "Your body interprets a lack of essential nutrients as yet another form of famine. When we finally do eat things containing the nutrients our bodies are starving for on a daily basis, our bodies get the message, 'OK. I'm not starving anymore. I don't need this fat anymore. It's safe to be thin now.'"

For me, when I began focusing more on nutrition, I decided that I wouldn't eat it if my great grandmother Rosa hadn't eaten it. She could do headstands in her 80s and was passionate about using food as medicine. If I'd given her a Slim-Fast shake and told her it was lunch, she would have looked at me like I was crazy.

As you use tapping to get in touch with what your body needs to be truly healthy, here are some general guidelines to consider:

**Listen to what your body is trying to tell you.** Start noticing how your body feels after a meal. Do you feel energized or are you experiencing symptoms like heartburn? Notice how you feel an hour after a meal. Did the food cause your energy to crash after a while? Become curious and be your own investigator to figure out what works best for you and your body.

**Slow down, and notice when your body *feels* full.** We live in a world where food is the most abundant it's ever been, but too often we forget that. When we're used to dieting and depriving ourselves, we eat quickly and consume more than the body needs and wants out of fear that we won't be able to have more later.

As Brian Wansink shares in *Mindless Eating*, the idea that we have to clean our plates disconnects us from the body. Rather than paying attention to signals the body may be giving us, the "clean plate mentality" encourages us to "dish it out, space out, and eat until it's gone."

Instead of worrying about finishing what's on your plate, stop just as you're beginning to feel satisfied. It's generally accepted that the body and brain need about 20 minutes to figure out whether we're full, so eating until you actually feel full will leave you overstuffed. Remember, you can always have more later when your body is truly hungry again.

**Go for quality.** When it comes to choosing quality food that provides our bodies with the most nutrients, Dr. Mark Hyman says it best in *The Blood Sugar Solution*:

> The take-home message is that the *quality of the food* we put in our bodies drives our gene function, metabolism, and health. It is not simply a matter of your weight, or calories in/calories out. Eating powerful, gene-altering, whole, real, fresh food that you cook yourself can rapidly change your biology . . . not starving yourself.

Dr. Hyman calls himself a "qualitarian." I like to think of myself the same way. For me that means choosing the freshest and highest-quality food I can find at any given moment. When I'm at home, that's easier. When I'm traveling, I prepare healthy snacks ahead of time but then also make some compromises, which I do without guilt or shame. Wherever I am, I do my best to choose the highest-quality options I can. That's enough to keep my body healthy and feeling great.

If I'm going to indulge in a sweet treat, I don't grab something from the gas station. Instead, I search out the real thing, like real chocolate in its purest form. When I have some, I take time to be present and really enjoy it. I love chocolate!

**Get in the kitchen (and make cooking fun!).** Your food should be made in a kitchen, not a lab. Grab your cookbooks; get your kids, spouse, partner, or friends involved; and make cooking fun again. Try new recipes that call for tons of fresh ingredients and perhaps new herbs and spices you haven't typically used. Make delicious food your latest and greatest adventure!

Excited about traveling to a certain part of the world? Pick recipes local to the region that use lots of fresh ingredients, and create an exotic adventure in your own kitchen.

If you're a salad fan, try adding fresh ingredients that are in season. It's a fun way to introduce variety into your bowl throughout the year.

Whatever you're planning to eat, do as much as you can to make preparing and cooking food enjoyable.

**Make it convenient.** If you fail to plan, you plan to fail. Junk food is so convenient, and most of us live fast-paced, super-busy lives. We need to make healthy eating convenient by preparing ahead of time. Every Sunday I spend some time cutting up fresh vegetables and storing them in the fridge, so I can quickly add them to my salads throughout the workweek.

Whether it means preparing your lunches the night before, meal planning for one week at a time, or creating grocery shopping lists for yourself or your family, take some time to plan ahead so healthy and wholesome eating is both tasty and convenient.

### When Real, Wholesome Food Seems Too Expensive

When I took classes in digital journalism in New York City, I was living with two other girls in a small apartment. *The Tapping Solution* documentary film hadn't had much success yet, and after paying for classes and my basic living expenses, I barely had any money left. I quickly realized that the only way I could eat healthfully was to plan ahead and buy food only at the grocery store. While a slice of pizza cost only a dollar, it wasn't aligned with my goals. I wanted to have energy and feel great. By choosing my food purchases carefully, I found that even in New York, I was able to afford healthy foods and stay within my budget. Planning ahead was key.

For resources on how to eat healthy on a budget go to www.TheTapping Solution.com/chapter10.

## The Myth of the Perfect Diet

I'd like to take this moment to apologize to all my friends and family for lecturing them every time I found the "perfect" diet. Each time, that new diet became my new religion and anyone not following the rules was sinning. As the religion's most fervent preacher, it was my job to lecture everyone and save them. Let's be honest—I was annoying.

When we are running the pattern of panic that we addressed earlier in this process, it's easy to get trapped in the mentality that there is some secret diet that will solve all our problems. We want to learn the one secret fruit that burns belly fat. We want to know exactly what we should eat and at what time in order to see a physical difference within 24 hours. That panic creates unrealistic expectations and robs us of the body's wisdom as well as our own common sense.

Some people have a foolish way of not minding, or pretending not to mind, what they eat. For my part, I mind my belly very studiously, and very carefully; for I look upon it, that he who does not mind his belly, will hardly mind anything else.

—SAMUEL JOHNSON

We've seen how damaging extreme dieting is to our emotions and our relationship with food. Eating as little food as possible also puts the body into starvation mode, which causes the body to hold on to fat because it doesn't know when the next meal will be. If we don't fully address how the pattern of panic affects our relationship with food, food soon becomes scary, even when we're focused on eating wholesome and nourishing food.

Amy shared that she became so health conscious that she'd walk into the grocery store and feel panicked because everything she looked at seemed bad for her. There's no question that our current food landscape needs attention, and the more aware of it we are, the more we see just how harmful ignorance can be. That said, awareness shouldn't equal panic. We can't learn new habits and be resourceful and creative when we're overwhelmed with panic.

When we approach eating healthy with curiosity and excitement, we are able to see the abundance of foods and flavors there are. Nutritious doesn't mean boring.

We also see that there is no "perfect" diet. I still occasionally drink wine and indulge in chocolate. My brother Alex still occasionally eats cheese that he knows won't make him feel great. The point is not to obsess about always eating the perfect food but to be conscious and do our best to enjoy the freshest and highest-quality food we can.

That's why the guidelines at the end of Chapter 4 are so vital (see pages 75–76). By being present with our food we can really enjoy that chocolate instead of inhaling it because we are searching for a feeling. Even when we choose to eat something that isn't ideally suited to our body's health and well-being, we can be present, enjoy it, and then move on to making a healthy choice the next time we're hungry.

We need to become friends with food again. It's a relationship we need to spend time on and really invest in. When we go from obsessing about diet foods to eating foods that nourish us, from obsessing about losing weight to obsessing about learning how to thrive with better health, we enjoy the journey of discovering what is best for us.

## Food Shouldn't Just Be Fuel or Medicine—It's Also about Pleasure

As we create a new relationship with food, one of the healthiest and best choices we can make is to experience true pleasure from it. While many of the food products on the market are devoid of nutrition, food itself isn't the enemy. The issue is that we have lost touch with what real food is. As a result, we've unintentionally been starving the body of the nutrition it's begging for.

That said, I don't ever want to look at food as *just* fuel. I don't think anyone should. We've lived for thousands of years enjoying and celebrating food. We deserve to honor that tradition and savor every delicious bite!

I always try to experience as much pleasure from food as possible. That doesn't just mean making tasty salads. It also means that when I eat something decadent and full of sugar, I get to enjoy every bite. Thanks to tapping, shame and guilt are no longer on my plate. When my sister-in-law makes her delicious dark chocolate cake for special occasions, I enjoy my piece fully, without guilt or shame. It goes right through me, without leaving stress, emotional residue, or added weight behind.

That's the power of allowing ourselves to experience pleasure from food, including occasional indulgences. And as we'll see in the next chapter, when we feel pleasure, our bodies can function at the highest level, supporting us as we support them.

# Creating a New Relationship with Food

**Karate Chop:** Even though I feel this panic around what I should and shouldn't eat, I choose to relax and trust my intuition. (*Repeat three times.*)

**Eyebrow:** All this panic around food . . .

**Side of Eye:** I don't know what I should eat.

**Under Eye:** I'm confused and stressed around food.

**Under Nose:** Everyone seems to disagree over the "right" way.

**Chin:** Can someone just tell me exactly what to eat?

**Collarbone:** This panic around food . . .

**Under Arm:** This panic to find the perfect diet . . .

**Top of Head:** This stress around what I eat . . .

**Eyebrow:** Food has become the enemy.

**Side of Eye:** I don't know what I should eat.

**Under Eye:** This stress leads me to my comfort food . . .

**Under Nose:** And then I panic about not eating "perfectly."

**Chin:** This back and forth . . .

**Collarbone:** I either eat perfectly . . .

**Under Arm:** Or I'm a mess.

**Top of Head:** This food anxiety . . .

**Eyebrow:** I've given away my power . . .

**Side of Eye:** To decide what's right for me.

**Under Eye:** Maybe there is no answer . . .

**Under Nose:** Maybe there is no perfect diet . . .

**Chin:** I'm open to seeing this in a new way.

**Collarbone:** Food isn't the enemy.

**Under Arm:** I choose to bring peace to this relationship.

**Top of Head:** I trust my body and do my best.

**Eyebrow:** As I let go of this panic now . . .

**Side of Eye:** I feel calm and confident.

**Under Eye:** As I let go of this search for the "perfect" diet . . .

**Under Nose:** I can notice what my body needs.

**Chin:** I begin to trust my intuition to lead me . . .

**Collarbone:** To information that can support me.

**Under Arm:** I naturally move away from diet foods . . .

**Top of Head:** And become attracted to information and foods that help my body thrive.

**Eyebrow:** I allow myself to experiment . . .

**Side of Eye:** To discover what is right for me.

**Under Eye:** I notice how my body reacts to certain foods.

**Under Nose:** I'm patient and curious.

**Chin:** There is no place to arrive to . . .

**Collarbone:** I'm constantly learning what my body needs . . .

**Under Arm:** And my body's needs are always changing.

**Top of Head:** I create a loving relationship with my body and food.

**Eyebrow:** I find ways to make my food more pleasurable.

**Side of Eye:** I'm open to trying new things.

**Under Eye:** I find joy in foods that nourish me . . .

**Under Nose:** And find the balance with indulgent food.

**Chin:** I can eat whatever I want . . .

**Collarbone:** And I choose what's right for me.

**Under Arm:** I stay open, patient, and curious . . .

**Top of Head:** As I become attracted to foods that help me thrive.

# Chapter 11

# Self-Care and Pleasure

So far we have learned about the consequences of stress, negative emotions, and limiting beliefs on our hormones, overall health, and weight. Now it's time to look at the other end of the spectrum—happiness.

Happiness creates a different set of internal circumstances. As I've been saying throughout the book: weight loss is not the key to happiness; it's the other way around. When we make our own happiness a priority, we can create a new relationship with the body we have and create an internal environment that supports weight loss. More important, when we experience more happiness, our lives open up in new and amazing ways.

## Happiness: The Weight Loss Drug

Like stress, happiness floods our bodies with hormones. The difference is that the hormones released by happiness and pleasure promote better health, improve digestion, increase metabolism, and even lengthen our life spans. Dr. Lissa Rankin, M.D., discusses the impact of happiness on health and well-being in her *New York Times* best-selling book, *Mind Over Medicine*:

People with higher levels of "subjective well-being" live up to ten years longer than those who don't. Happiness also affects some health outcomes, including success rates of stem-cell transplantation, control of diabetes, rates of full-blown AIDS in HIV-positive patients, and recovery from stroke, heart surgery, and hip fracture.

She goes on to add:

Studies show that positive psychological states, such as joy, happiness, and positive energy, as well as characteristics such as life satisfaction, hopefulness, optimism, and a sense of humor, result in lower mortality rates and extended longevity in both healthy and diseased populations. In fact, happiness and related mental states reduce the risk or limit the severity of heart disease, lung disease, diabetes, hypertension, and colds. According to a Dutch study of elderly patients, upbeat mental states reduced an individual's risk of death by 50 percent over the study's nine-year duration.

While we may be excited to learn that happiness, the natural outcome of pleasure, improves our overall health, the question remains: how does pleasure impact weight?

> . . . pleasure is a powerful metabolizer that increases oxygenation and blood flow and decreases the production of cortisol and insulin, ultimately helping to burn fat and build muscle.
>
> —MARC DAVID

Sally, one of my online students, experienced the power of pleasure during a two-week vacation in Italy. During her trip she continued tapping and also made sure to enjoy some special treats, including her first sfogliatelle, a cone-shaped filled pastry, in Naples. When she returned home from the trip, Sally noticed that her clothes felt looser. Much to her surprise, she had lost seven pounds!

Most of us hear stories like that and wonder how they're possible. We assume we're missing information or being misled in some way. That's because we haven't been taught how crucial pleasure is to weight loss, as well as to overall health and well-being.

In *The Slow Down Diet* Marc David discusses the vacation weight loss phenomenon, which is an experience many people have at some point. Even while indulging in richer foods than they eat at home, they come home lighter than before they left. "Remove vitamin P, pleasure," he writes, "and the nutritional value of our food plummets. Add vitamin P and your meal is metabolically optimized."

He goes on to explain how endorphins, the body's pleasure chemicals, impact metabolism and weight loss:

> What's most unusual about the endorphins is that not only are they molecules of pleasure, but they also stimulate fat mobilization. In other words, the same chemical that makes you feel good burns body fat. Furthermore, the greater the endorphin release in your digestive tract, the more blood and oxygen will be delivered there. This means increased digestion, assimilation, and ultimately greater efficiency in calorie burning.

## What Happens When We Relax

If relaxation and pleasure are so good for our health, why aren't they priorities in our lives?

The reality is that we live in a culture that values speed and productivity, so relaxation often gets a bad rap. We're taught that taking time to sit outside means we're lazy and unproductive; solutions to problems come through hard work, not relaxation. As a result, when we're stressed and overwhelmed, we often limit or cut out all forms of pleasure and self-care except food. We rely on stress and worry to carry us through even though they can damage our health and well-being.

When we look at what happens when we relax, we see how important it is to our health and well-being, as well as the flow of our lives. Think for a moment how often you've gotten your best ideas while in the shower. That's because water is relaxing, so the brain can solve problems in the bath or shower that it can't solve when you're under stress.

The same is true of taking a walk. We've already seen that many of the greatest minds in history have relied on walks as a way to boost their creativity, solve problems, and live more productive lives. That's because walking is pleasurable and relaxing, so it allows us to think better and be more effective.

Tapping has a very similar relaxing effect, of course, and it allows us to get in touch with our intuition and access the solutions that are all around us and inside us. That's why we at The Tapping Solution regularly get hundreds of e-mails about Aha! moments people have while tapping.

## Why We Don't Make Pleasure a Priority

While it's true that our culture discounts the importance of relaxation and pleasure, often the real reasons we deny ourselves self-care and pleasure are less obvious than we realize. Although we may blame our lack of self-care and pleasure on our fast-paced lives, or perhaps on a shortage of time and/or money, when we dig deeper we discover that deeply ingrained cultural beliefs about our value as women have been holding us back.

Looking back through history, our culture has been dominated by the belief that women are less valuable than men. For thousands of years, our value as women has been measured *only* by our ability to nurture others. While we are natural caretakers who do love to nurture others, it has only been very recently that our other gifts—our intellect, creativity, and much more—have been recognized as valuable. Because we have always wanted to be valuable and contribute to society, we learned a very long time ago that we should spend all of our time and energy caring for others. Taking time for self-care and pleasure, then, became something we shouldn't do because it decreased our value as women and as caretakers.

While I don't believe in using this cultural heritage to blame men or make ourselves victims, I do think it's important that we acknowledge this societal programming because during this journey, most women run into a lot of resistance around self-care. We need to understand that countless generations of women have been taught that self-sacrifice makes us better and that self-care and pleasure make us selfish and wrong.

These ideas tend to be passed down from one generation to the next in ways that are both conscious and unconscious. Often, we're taught to sacrifice ourselves for the sake of others in incredibly subtle ways. I love the way my friend Regena Thomashauer, who runs Mama Gena's School of Womanly Arts, explained it to me one day. She said, "Our mothers never sat us down and said, 'Baby, darling, it is a privilege to be a woman and the best thing that you can do is learn what pleasures you, what lights you up and excites you.'"

Because we haven't been taught to appreciate and love ourselves in this way, we don't feel like we deserve self-care and pleasure. Instead, we cling to our To Do lists and sacrifice our health and well-being for the sake of others. Then, when we feel deprived of our basic human need for relaxation and enjoyment, we turn to food as our sole source of pleasure. When we then try to deprive ourselves of food through dieting, we deny the last bit of pleasure we have in our lives. And that strategy never works!

Body confidence, weight loss, and better health are about understanding that we deserve self-care and pleasure and that our value extends far beyond our ability to care for others. Self-care and pleasure are, in fact, basic requirements for our well-being. Only when we truly believe that can we seek out healthier and more fulfilling ways to feel good will we be able to lose the weight and gain confidence in ourselves.

# The Real Reason for Self-Care and Pleasure

We've all heard it said that we can't take care of others if we don't take care of ourselves. That's a socially acceptable reason for self-care because it reinforces the idea that our value lies in our caretaking abilities. It also happens to be true. When we skip self-care, we burn out, and when we burn out, everyone and everything in our lives suffers.

What we realize when we prioritize self-care and pleasure in our daily lives, though, is that it's about a lot more than being better able to help others. During an interview I did with Cheryl Richardson, best-selling author of *The Art of Extreme Self-Care*, she made a very powerful point about the real reason we need to practice self-care. Here's what she shared:

> The acceptable thing for me to say is, honey, if you take better care of yourself, then that means you'll be a better person to be around. While that's true, what I really want to say as I've gotten older is, honey, if you take better care of yourself, the negative self-talk is going to stop. Honey, if you take better care of yourself, you're going to feel stronger in your body. Honey, if you take better care of yourself, you're going to care more about what you think and less about what other people think. And then you're going to be more powerful in the world. You're going to effect change in your life and in the lives of the people around you. You're going to have a huge impact on the planet because one of the ways that women sit on their power is by not taking care of their bodies.

I was almost stunned into silence by these words. Although I had practiced and even preached self-care, it didn't hit me until that moment just how incredibly vital it is. It's not until we make a practice of connecting with ourselves on a regular and frequent basis that we can dim our negative self-talk and truly appreciate ourselves. Only then can we feel confident and beautiful in our own skin. Only then can we step into our power and live our dreams. Self-care can't be looked at as a luxury; it's a necessity.

# Why We Avoid Self-Care and Pleasure

While the practice of self-care and pleasure may quiet our negative self-talk, that same negative self-talk is often the biggest reason we deny ourselves self-care and pleasure.

When we have spent so many years denying pleasure and hating the body we have, spending quiet time alone is often when our negative self-talk is at its worst. That makes self-care and pleasure feel unpleasant, even painful.

Speaking to my friend Kelly, who has three young children, I was reminded of how difficult it can be to reintroduce self-care into our lives. She called me one day while her kids were napping and casually mentioned how tired she felt. When I suggested she lie down for a bit, she said she couldn't. "Every time I try to nap, all I hear is my dad's voice telling me to stop being useless," she explained. She knew she needed the extra sleep, but she couldn't get the memory of her dad's words out of her head.

So many of us have had some version of that same experience: we want to take the time for ourselves but then struggle to quiet the negative self-talk or other critical voices in our heads. At those times it often feels easier to seek out a distraction like food, television, or the Internet than to face our self-talk and the emotions it creates. When we give a voice to those emotions while we tap, we can learn to truly enjoy self-care and relaxation.

Is there a voice telling you that you're doing something wrong when you're eating slowly and being present with your food, sitting outside, or taking a nap? Tap while you express that voice to release its power over you.

As we add self-care and pleasure back into our lives, we also need to remember that self-care takes practice. Even after tapping, it may feel like a foreign experience. Allow yourself to experiment with new ways to relax, and feel free to refer to the list of different kinds of self-care at the end of this chapter (pages 237–239).

Let's do some tapping now on quieting the negative self-talk so you can enjoy self-care. When you think about taking time for yourself, what voice comes up? Is there a particular emotion or sensation in your body that accompanies that voice? Write down your answers and measure the intensity of that voice, emotion, or feeling in your body on a scale of 0 to 10. That becomes your tapping target. This tapping script may help.

**Karate Chop:** Even though I hear this critical voice when I try to relax, I love and accept myself. (*Repeat three times.*)

**Eyebrow:** This voice that I hear when I try to relax . . .

**Side of Eye:** It tells me, "Stop being lazy."

**Under Eye:** "Work harder."

**Under Nose:** "Go make something of yourself."

**Chin:** "Stop being selfish."

**Collarbone:** "Do something constructive."

**Under Arm:** "You should be further along than this."

**Top of Head:** "Keep pushing."

*When the intensity of your initial tapping target is 5 or lower, you can move on to the positive.*

**Eyebrow:** I was given the gift of this life . . .

**Side of Eye:** And I honor it by enjoying it.

**Under Eye:** As I take care of myself, I see my true value.

**Under Nose:** Self-care is an essential way . . .

**Chin:** To discover my power.

**Collarbone:** As I replenish my resources, I can shine my light.

**Under Arm:** As I relax, answers become clear.

**Top of Head:** It feels so good to feel good.

*Take a deep breath and check in with how you feel. Measure the*
*intensity again and continue tapping until you experience relief.*

# The Hidden Rules in Your Head

While tapping through resistance to self-care and pleasure, many of us
also realize that in addition to negative self-talk, we've created limiting
rules about when and why we're allowed to take care of ourselves and
feel happy. Because these rules have become so ingrained, we often
forget to notice them.

While tapping, Kavita realized that her happiness had always been
dependent on her family. If they weren't happy, she couldn't be happy;
and if her children didn't behave in a certain way, she felt she needed
to punish herself for not being a good enough mother. Another client,
Doreen, didn't feel she could be happy or take care of herself until all
of her son's needs were met. Because he had severe autism, that meant
putting her happiness on hold until there was a cure. And there's
always that old standby: we can't be happy or feel confident in our
body until we lose the weight.

Too often, the rules we've created around our right to experience
happiness make self-care and pleasure difficult, even impossible. When
we're able to see these rules for what they are—excuses for depriving ourselves of self-care and pleasure—we realize that we alone are
responsible for our own happiness. Only we can decide that we're worthy of good things. Making other people responsible for our happiness
puts an unfair burden on them and drains us. Being responsible for
other people's happiness creates an equal burden and stress.

To begin breaking this cycle, you need to disconnect from these
rules and create healthy boundaries around your own happiness. As
part of that process, imagine talking to your spouse or a family member you've tried to make happy. This is a different process of simply
tapping and talking. You don't ever need to say these words to that
person; just imagine saying them. You can focus your tapping on one
point or move to another point with every sentence. Notice if you can

say these words and feel calm and peaceful. Tap through the points while saying this out loud:

> I am only responsible for my own happiness. I love you, but it's not my job to make you happy. The truth is that I can't make you or anyone else happy; I can only make myself happy. Happiness is a choice and each of us can choose it or not. Loving and supporting you doesn't mean I need to fix you. I have faith in your abilities and in your spiritual journey. I trust that you will make the right decisions for you. I let go of the need to make you happy. I choose to be happy now and love you.

## Carrying the Weight of the World

As naturally intuitive, compassionate, and caring people, we often feel other people's pain, and then we allow ourselves to feel responsible for their happiness. When we feel like we have to be martyrs and carry the weight of the world on our shoulders, that weight may physically appear on the body.

While our intentions may be loving, we need to understand that our ability to feel compassion doesn't mean that we need to take on other people's pain. We're not helping ourselves or anyone else by overgiving. Feeling hurt when someone else feels hurt doesn't lessen their pain. Being angry when someone else is angry doesn't lead to a resolution.

The world doesn't need us to be martyrs. The world needs our gifts. It needs our intelligence, our laughter, and yes, our love, but not love that looks and feels like self-sacrifice. The world needs us to take care of ourselves so we can shine brightly and inspire others to do the

> The world needs our gifts. It needs our intelligence, our laughter, and yes, our love, but not love that looks and feels like self-sacrifice.
>
> —JESSICA ORTNER

same. And again, we can't give others what we ourselves don't have. We can't spread peace, love, or hope if we haven't experienced those things ourselves.

## Have Faith in Others' Journeys

As we begin setting healthy boundaries and stop taking on other people's pain, we sometimes need to let go and have faith that the people we love will find their own way. I learned that lesson with a friend of mine. Whenever I saw her struggling and suffering, I jumped in to try to help, but the more I tried to help, the more she retreated. She didn't want my help.

Over time I learned to question my own intentions, and I realized that by jumping in to solve her problems, I had violated her boundaries. *Who am I to pretend I know the answer for her?* I wondered. *How can I pretend to know how she should live her life?* As I let go of the idea that her life should be a certain way, I began to trust that she could handle her own journey. It wasn't always easy. Many times I found myself wanting to "save" her from the pain I'd been through, but then I'd remind myself that the best way I could support her was to have faith in her ability and simply let her know I was there for her if she needed me.

When we let go of how we think people "should" behave and how the world "should" be, we can let go of the weight of the world. This only happens when we have faith in something greater than ourselves. We can't be the master of the universe; we can only learn to dance with the ever-changing beat and do our best to enjoy ourselves. The more we try to "fix" things, the more we run ourselves into the ground. In the moment, we can never know the greater picture, but we can still trust that things will work out. Some of the hardest times in my life ended up being the biggest blessings because I learned so much from them. When we allow ourselves to really see the value of our challenges, we can have faith in other people's ability to undergo similar experiences. We can support them without asking them to behave in a way that satisfies our own needs or desires.

When we are able to truly trust, we unburden ourselves and other people in a healthy and loving way that also allows us to take better care of ourselves, not just physically but emotionally and spiritually as well. The lightness we feel in spirit then begins to show up on the body.

## The Power of No

When Ann, a registered nursing assistant, first heard her voice mail message, her stomach dropped. She had missed the call while swimming after work, which was the result of her intention to take more time for self-care. The call she had missed was a request from her office to come into work on her day off. After listening to it, she felt conflicted. While she could use the money and had always said yes when people needed her, she also felt that she needed time for herself.

After doing some tapping, Ann realized that she needed to take her scheduled day off. Feeling nervous about saying no, she tapped again before returning the call and then gracefully explained that she wouldn't be able to come in on that day. The office secretary responded, "Oh Ann, you're breaking my heart." To her surprise Ann replied, "Sorry I can't help. I'm sure it will work out."

Ann was shocked when she hung up the phone. She couldn't believe she had stood her ground. But as doubts began to creep in, she repeated the words "Oh Ann, you're breaking my heart" while tapping. She said those words until they no longer triggered her in any way. She felt proud of herself for saying no.

Ann hadn't made any plans for her day off, but after she said no to working that day, a friend invited her on a sunset cruise. Because she'd succeeded in preserving her day off, Ann was able to say yes to a fun and pleasurable experience. Her body was soon coursing with healthy hormones!

Like Ann, many other clients share that they feel like they can't say no to requests, even when saying yes comes at the expense of their health and well-being. For me the fear of saying no showed up in an unexpected way. I was afraid that if I lost weight, and as a result became successful (at this time I still believed that being thin meant I

## When People Respond Negatively to Healthy Boundaries

There are times when people may not respond positively to us when we say no. If this is a pattern, it may be time to consider the kinds of people we're surrounding ourselves with. Some people may be "toxic" for us. They won't support our healthy boundaries and our need to care for ourselves because it threatens them in some way. In those cases, we need to think about whether they're a healthy part of our lives or if we need to distance ourselves from them in some way.

At other times, those same people just need time to adjust to our new way of behaving. When you make a change, you may kick up some dust. Give the dust some time to settle. It may take time for others to adjust to your new pattern of creating healthy boundaries.

would be successful), life would change. Not being able to say no created a fear of success. I worried that if I went for my dreams, things would move too fast. I was afraid of getting overwhelmed and not being able to keep up.

When we don't know how to create healthy boundaries by saying no, parking ourselves in front of the TV with a box of cookies often feels safer than going for what we want and need. Because we don't feel we can say no, going for our dreams, however big or small, can feel like driving at full speed without brakes. When we crash, we turn to food once again, this time hoping to soften the blow while complaining about the unfairness of it all. After all, we tried *so hard* and look what happened.

If we are not able to say no in the first place, we've set ourselves up for failure and burnout. When we allow ourselves to use that brake and say no, we can slow down, stop, and when needed, change directions. We no longer need to turn to food for relief because we feel more in control of our lives.

While we may fear that saying no will lessen our success and damage our relationships, we often find, as I did, that the opposite is true. When we can say no in a positive and caring way, we're able to replenish ourselves and shine our own light.

## Learning to Say No

Saying no when we need to replenish ourselves is something that most of us, including me, continue to work on, even once we've seen how powerful it is. For me, when I'm uncertain about something, it's easy to fall back into my old "good girl" pattern of saying yes to please others. It happens less often now than it used to, but when I do catch myself being that "good girl," I give myself permission to change my mind and say no instead.

To help you say no when you feel you need to, here are some great tips from Cheryl Richardson's *The Art of Extreme Self-Care* on how to respond to requests:

- **Buy some time.** Instead of immediately saying yes, gently let them know you'll get back to them.

- **Do a gut check.** Giving yourself some time to think gives you a chance to check in with yourself and figure out what's the best answer for you.

- **Tell the truth directly—with grace and love.** When it's time to say no, make sure to be honest while also being loving and gracious. Express your appreciation and thanks for the invitation or offer you were given, and then be honest about why it doesn't work for you. You don't need to go into extreme detail with your explanation; just give them a reason why you can't say yes.

Let's do some tapping now on learning to say no.

Imagine a friend, co-worker, or family member asking for something. They need your help but you know that saying yes is going to be very taxing on your emotional and physical health. Imagine saying, "No, I'm sorry I can't help you this time." Does that create any panic in your body? Does any emotion or belief come up when you imagine yourself saying no? Take note of those feelings and thoughts and write down their intensity on a scale of 0 to 10.

> **Karate Chop:** Even though I feel this panic at the thought of saying no, I love and accept myself. (*Repeat three times.*)
>
> **Eyebrow:** I can't say no.
>
> **Side of Eye:** Part of me really wants to say no.
>
> **Under Eye:** Part of me wants to say yes.
>
> **Under Nose:** I like saying yes, but I'm burned out.
>
> **Chin:** I want to be helpful but not at the expense of my health.

**Collarbone:** Finding balance by saying no.

**Under Arm:** But what if they get mad at me?

**Top of Head:** I give a voice to my fears now.

*Continue expressing your fears around saying no while you tap. Get specific. Are you scared of their response? What scenario are you playing in your mind? Continue tapping as you get clearer. When the emotional intensity is 5 or lower, begin incorporating these positive tapping statements.*

**Eyebrow:** If it's not a clear yes, then it's a no.

**Side of Eye:** I begin to care more about what I think.

**Under Eye:** I find a graceful way to say no.

**Under Nose:** This is easier than I thought.

**Chin:** The more I respect my time . . .

**Collarbone:** The more others respect my time.

## What Happened When I Stopped Being a Yes-a-holic

While I'm often outspoken, I've never felt comfortable with conflict so have often gone out of my way to avoid it. For years that meant always saying yes, even when it drained me. Saying no felt too scary because I thought people would get angry with me. I also thought that if I said no, other people wouldn't see me as valuable.

What happened as a result of me being a yes-a-holic was typical. I burned out and began to resent the people I loved.

**Under Arm:** As I say no to someone else . . .

**Top of Head:** I say yes to myself.

*Take a deep breath and check in with how you feel. Measure the intensity again and continue tapping until you experience relief.*

## The Cycle of Guilt and Resentment

Evelyn is a single mother of a five-year-old and a full-time social worker who lives with her elderly parents on their farm because her dad is in a wheelchair and needs more help than her mother can provide. She is also responsible for taking care of the many animals on the farm. When Evelyn says she doesn't have time for self-care, even I hesitate to argue with her!

Understandably, when she began my class Evelyn felt exhausted and depleted. In the rare moments when she could stop and relax, she became overwhelmed with guilt, thinking of all the things she needed to get done. She felt resentful of the people she loved and then guilty for feeling resentful.

After tapping through my fear and limiting beliefs about how others would react to me saying no, I slowly began trying it out. It felt awkward and uncomfortable at first, but what happened over a bit of time was pretty amazing.

First of all, none of my fears came true. No one got mad at me, and instead of becoming less valuable, people began valuing my time more. Because I was only saying yes when I really meant it, I was also more present in everything I was doing. As a result, new opportunities began appearing. In setting healthy boundaries for myself by saying no when I needed to, I began saying yes to myself and the life I truly wanted.

As much as Evelyn disliked having these feelings, she couldn't seem to find her way out of the cycle of guilt about not doing more and resentment when she did. She loved her family and her job and wanted to be able to enjoy her life. When she began tapping for 10 to 15 minutes a day during the course, she realized that in fact she could make some time for herself each day; even a few minutes here and there added up.

As she tapped on a regular basis, she was surprised to realize how much negative self-talk she was experiencing, and she used tapping to

## "I Don't Have Time and/or Money" Means It's Time to Increase Self-Care

The more stressed and stretched we feel, the more self-care we need. Cindy realized this after tapping on why she "didn't have time" to take care of herself anymore. She had gone out of her way to tend to her health, meditate, go to church, and do yoga until she became a mom—and all of that stopped. Suddenly her children were her first priority, and work came second. Self-care had almost completely dropped off her schedule. She just couldn't find the time.

When she tapped, she realized she needed to find a way to make self-care a priority again. Now when she drops off her daughter at the school bus, she takes a 20-minute walk and then spends some time tapping or meditating before starting work. Since making self-care a priority, she's been shocked to notice that her business has picked up. "I really think the reason I'm making more money now is that I am *finally* listening to my inner voice and taking care of me," she shared.

When we focus on pleasure and happiness and make self-care a priority, we often find that we experience our lives differently and new opportunities appear.

quiet it. Since then, Evelyn has made self-care and pleasure a regular part of her days. In addition to tapping and meditating each day, she checks in with herself throughout the day, doing a few rounds of tapping in the bathroom at work whenever she's feeling overwhelmed. She also makes a point of simply sitting on the front porch to enjoy gazing out at nature. She could never have these serene moments before because of her negative self-talk and guilt.

As a result of her willingness to incorporate self-care and pleasure into her daily life, Evelyn has developed a new appreciation for her body. "I feel like I'm worthy and much more self-confident," she shared. "Before, when I had a brief moment of liking me, it was because I had on a new outfit or was having a great hair day—it was all on the surface. Now it's a more gentle and wholesome feeling of gratitude toward myself. The really cool part is that I see that same gentle kindness coming out in my daughter."

Not long after she incorporated self-care into her daily life, Evelyn shared that she was able to detach completely from her old cycle of guilt and resentment. As a result, she felt an even closer connection with her daughter and parents. The weight was coming off, too, without her feeling like she had to work at it. She was thrilled and amazed by the difference her new habit of self-care and pleasure was making throughout her life.

## Asking for Help

Too many of us have been tricked into believing that being strong, independent women means we need to do everything ourselves. When we take on too much and don't ask for help, we tell ourselves that we're doing as we should. If we just push ourselves to give more, surely someone will notice and we'll finally receive the love we've felt deprived of. Instead, because we're unwilling to ask for the support we need, we start and end our days feeling exhausted and unloved because no one has bothered to notice how much help we need.

The truth is that we won't receive the support we need until we ask for it. Just because we can do it all doesn't mean we should. And when we don't speak up about our needs, we're asking our loved ones to read our minds—and then we resent them when they fail our test. By not being open and honest about the support we need, we're selling ourselves short and setting our relationships up for failure.

Being a strong woman is very important to me. But doing it all on my own is not.

—REBA MCENTIRE

Finally allowing ourselves to practice self-care and feel pleasure enables us to see that in pushing ourselves so hard to be "good enough," we've created blocks to receiving the love that others feel for us and the support they want to give us. Often, we judge ourselves when we even *think* about asking for help. The key isn't to never help anyone else and always say no.

Wanting to help others is a beautiful thing, but we do need to know our boundaries and ask for help when we need it. As much as we give, we need to find balance by being able to ask for and receive the love and support we need in return. If we don't, we find ourselves helping others and then feeling resentful of them instead of feeling more connected to them.

There's a brilliant video of Brené Brown speaking to Oprah on Oprah.com. In it she says, "When you cannot accept and ask for help without self-judgment, then when you offer other people help you are always doing so with judgment because you have attached judgment with asking for help." She continued, "When you think *I'm helping you because one day I'll need help,* that's connection."

Let's do some tapping now to release the judgment so we can experience more balance and connection through giving and receiving help.

Imagine yourself asking for help. Maybe it's something you need help with right now. When you imagine asking, do you feel any tension in your body? Any strong emotions? Any disempowering thoughts? Take note of them and measure their intensity on a scale of 0 to 10. Begin tapping as you focus on your answers. This tapping script may help you.

**Karate Chop:** Even though I have this anxiety around asking for help, I love and accept myself. (*Repeat three times.*)

**Eyebrow:** I can't ask for help.

**Side of Eye:** It feels wrong.

**Under Eye:** I have to do it all to prove I'm enough.

**Under Nose:** To be a strong, intelligent woman . . .

**Chin:** I should be able to do it all myself.

**Collarbone:** To ask for help is to admit failure.

**Under Arm:** Is this really true?

**Top of Head:** These stories I've been telling myself . . .

**Eyebrow:** These fears around asking for help . . .

**Side of Eye:** What if they say no?

**Under Eye:** What if I'm a burden on them?

**Under Nose:** It's okay if they say no.

**Chin:** The same way it's okay if I say no.

**Collarbone:** I am calm and clear.

**Under Arm:** It's safe to receive help . . .

**Top of Head:** The same way I give help.

*Take a deep breath and check in with how you feel. Measure the intensity again and continue tapping until you experience relief.*

# How Self-Care Is Easy and Valuable

When I share self-care tips with students and clients, they're often hesitant and skeptical at first. "Pleasure is too easy, and self-care is too selfish," they may say or just think to themselves. Until they do some tapping and try practicing self-care, the benefits of pleasure don't compute.

> Caring for myself is not self-indulgence, it is self-preservation.
>
> —AUDRE LORDE

I understand that. Many of us, including me, have had the limiting belief that when something isn't hard, it isn't valuable. We have spent years mastering the art of feeling overwhelmed, convinced that we have no choice but to feel consumed by stress. Over time feeling overwhelmed has become an ingrained habit. It's how we live our lives.

When we tap and let go of the feeling that supported our habit of always being overwhelmed, the habit may still be in place. Habits are easier to change once we've cleared the negative emotion that fueled them, but to break a habit completely, we often need to take action.

When it comes to pleasure and self-care, many of us are simply out of practice. To make it a daily habit, we may need to make a conscious effort to replace our old habit of stress with a new habit of self-care. Lucky for us, practicing pleasure is . . . well . . . pleasurable!

Happiness is directly linked to how much pleasure and self-care we allow ourselves to experience. It's time to stop pretending that other people can give us happiness and instead, give it to ourselves. "Because it makes me happy" is the most valid reason to do almost anything.

That leaves us with one last question: how can we begin practicing self-care and experiencing more pleasure? To answer that question, I'm sharing my favorite self-care tips. You'll find that these are simple ways to practice self-care. There is no struggle, and many of them are free as well. When it comes to pleasure, easy is often the best.

*Note:* If you find your mind resorting to worry, stress, and negative self-talk, take some time to tap on what's bothering you. By tapping first, you can retrain your mind to understand that it's okay to relax and enjoy yourself. Here are some of my tips for practicing more self-care and experiencing more pleasure:

**Differentiate between personal development and self-care.** First we need to understand that personal development and self-care are not always the same thing. While our desire to develop spiritually, emotionally, and physically is positive, personal development can also be hard work. Self-care is giving ourselves a break from the many different kinds of hard work we do. Learning how to improve ourselves is incredibly important and valuable, but when we practice self-care, we need to allow ourselves to relax the mind and be present in the body.

**Do nothing (or at least, very little).** We spend so much time and energy running around tending to our To Do lists that we forget to stop, even when we're exhausted and overwhelmed. Instead of trying to move faster and do more, take some time to experience nature and let your mind wander. You might cuddle your pet, do some knitting, color in your children's coloring books, soak your feet in warm water, or stare at your favorite painting. Try anything that feels relaxing—for no reason at all.

**Make your living environment more pleasurable.** Sometimes tiny changes, like a flower on your dining room table or desk, can make all the difference in how you feel. I often light a beautiful candle while I'm working. When I make my green juice, I drink it from a wineglass because it feels more pleasurable that way. Just by focusing on how to bring more pleasure into your everyday life, you will find yourself making little but important changes that make you feel good. Look at your living environment and ask yourself, *How can I make this space more pleasurable to be in?*

**Start a gratitude or pleasure journal.** We can get so busy that we forget to notice what we love about our lives. Make a habit of writing down what you're grateful for in a journal each night, and what brought you pleasure that day. Nothing is too small or big to write down, so whether it's a cool breeze or an endearing moment with a loved one, jot it down. It's a great way to bring more pleasure into your life and to notice how much pleasure and love you already have.

**Expand your joy bubble.** This is one of my favorite happiness exercises. Whenever you have a minute, whether you're walking, waiting somewhere, or doing something else, consciously think of something that brings you joy or makes you laugh or feel grateful. Focus on it and let yourself feel that positive feeling in your body, letting the energy of happiness expand there. For me, it feels almost like a warm bubble in my heart center, and as I focus on things that make me feel good, the bubble expands. Try it as often as you can. The more we're in that happy energy, the more amazing things tend to happen in our lives. After I began practicing this, I found a quote by Paramahansa Yogananda that explained what I was intuitively doing to feel more joy:

> When a little bubble of joy appears in your sea of consciousness, take hold of it and keep expanding it. Meditate on it, and it will grow larger. Keep puffing at the bubble until it breaks its confining walls and becomes a sea of joy.

**Put on that lipstick.** Taking time every day to put on clothes and makeup that make us feel good isn't vanity; it's an important way to care for ourselves and celebrate our beauty. We need to stop selling ourselves short by hiding under ill-fitting clothes and not taking time to do our hair. Spending five to ten minutes on your hair, makeup, and clothes each morning is often enough to change your energy throughout the entire day. When you see your own beauty, enhancing it is a way of expressing self-love and respect.

**Focus on sleep.** Too many of us aren't getting enough sleep, and it's time we made it a bigger priority. One thing I've found helpful is to figure out how long it actually takes me to get to bed. Between tapping, washing my face, and sometimes doing some yoga to relax, it takes me 75 to 90 minutes to get into bed. (I happily embrace my daily habit of what some people call "dilly dallying.") Knowing this helps me plan ahead and start early enough to get a good night's sleep.

It's also important to look at how you use your time at night. Studies show that the light from computer screens, digital reading devices, and televisions can interfere with sleep, so it's a good idea to turn off your television and shut down all digital devices at least an hour before you go to sleep. Instead, do some tapping, write in your gratitude and pleasure journal, or read a magazine or book.

Go here to listen to my tapping meditation for getting a restful night's sleep: www.TheTappingSolution.com/chapter11.

**Always see the magnificence in the mundane.** Throughout the day, look at what you're doing and ask, *How can I make this more pleasurable?* For me, cleaning the house is more pleasurable when I listen to an audio book. Standing in line at the grocery store is more pleasurable when I think about things that excite me.

Allow yourself to feel moved by a song on the radio, or look closely at a blade of grass and marvel at its beauty and strength. Be enthusiastic about something—anything! Notice how soothing it feels to hold a warm cup of tea in your hands. Stand outside, close your eyes, and lift your face to the sun and feel the warmth sink into your soul. Instead of just pushing your child on the swing, get on the swing yourself.

### Surfing the Internet Is a Distraction, Not Self-Care

Many women I work with share that they often spend time at night surfing the Internet and Facebook because they feel like they give so much to everyone else that they need some time to numb out.

Surfing the Internet is not self-care. It's a way of distracting ourselves that often increases stress and deprives us of quality time with ourselves. If you find yourself overgiving to others all day long, it's time to create healthy boundaries so you don't feel a need to numb out at the end of the day.

For some of us, disconnecting from technology can feel uncomfortable. Several years ago I did a social media and technology "detox" while traveling in China. It wasn't planned, and feeling disconnected from the social media world made me a bit anxious for the first few days—but after those first few days, I didn't miss it. In fact, I was able to enjoy the simple pleasures of daily life a lot more without constantly checking my phone and connecting to social media.

I now make a habit of occasionally doing a social media detox. When we focus on everyone else's lives, we have less time to cultivate our own. I sometimes block social media for entire weekends, and I highly recommend trying this periodically.

Slip into the swimming pool and be present with the sensation of the water swishing around your legs.

Being playful and silly doesn't lower your IQ. Being optimistic doesn't make you naïve. As women, we are dynamic. Sometimes we need to have serious business conversations, but that doesn't mean we can't let ourselves be carried away by positive emotions afterward.

When we use tapping to clear our blocks to self-care and pleasure and begin celebrating ourselves and the magnificence that surrounds us, we can finally notice and embrace the light and love that have always been all around us. That is when the true magic of transformation happens, not just in our hearts, but also in our bodies.

# Overcoming Blocks to Self-Care and Pleasure

**Karate Chop:** Even though I've had all this resistance to seeking pleasure, I love and accept myself and I'm okay. (*Repeat three times.*)

**Eyebrow:** It doesn't feel right to take time for myself.

**Side of Eye:** There is too much to do.

**Under Eye:** Too many people depend on me.

**Under Nose:** I just don't have the time.

**Chin:** All this fear around what might happen . . .

**Collarbone:** If I decide to take a break.

**Under Arm:** I care so deeply . . .

**Top of Head:** That I feel the need to worry.

**Eyebrow:** I just can't let go of control . . .

**Side of Eye:** And take a break.

**Under Eye:** I must keep going.

**Under Nose:** I must keep pushing.

**Chin:** That's what people value about me.

**Collarbone:** Is that really true?

**Under Arm:** This story I've been telling myself . . .

**Top of Head:** About why I can't take time for myself.

**Eyebrow:** I've been made to believe . . .

**Side of Eye:** That love means I need to worry . . .

**Under Eye:** That caring means I need to worry.

**Under Nose:** I can love and care deeply . . .

**Chin:** While letting go of this worry.

**Collarbone:** I have faith things will work out.

**Under Arm:** It is safe for me to relax . . .

**Top of Head:** And open my mind to the possibilities.

**Eyebrow:** It's safe to take time for me.

**Side of Eye:** As I begin to value my time . . .

**Under Eye:** Others begin to value my time.

**Under Nose:** As I say no to others . . .

**Chin:** I say yes to myself . . .

**Collarbone:** Yes to self-care . . .

**Under Arm:** Yes to pleasure . . .

**Top of Head:** Yes to joy.

**Eyebrow:** As I do this . . .

**Side of Eye:** Miracles appear in my life.

**Under Eye:** I notice all the support around me.

**Under Nose:** I begin to trust in life.

**Chin:** I begin to trust my inner voice.

**Collarbone:** I know what is right for me.

**Under Arm:** I choose to feel good for no reason . . .

**Top of Head:** And inspire others to do the same.

**Eyebrow:** I make pleasure easy.

**Side of Eye:** I don't need the perfect moment to feel good.

**Under Eye:** I choose to feel good now.

**Under Nose:** I release the need to make life hard to prove my value.

**Chin:** I now find ways to make life easy because I know my value.

**Collarbone:** It is safe for me to take time for myself.

**Under Arm:** It is safe to be happy for no reason.

**Top of Head:** It feels so good to feel good.

# Chapter 12

# The Journey Forward

"I finally feel comfortable in my body. I feel beautiful!" Celina shared during a live call in my class. She didn't feel like she needed to lose any more weight. She was healthy and finally able to appreciate her body.

Just as I was about to respond, she asked, "So I'm wondering . . . when am I done?"

"Done with what?" I asked.

We both laughed. "I don't actually know!" she said. "I guess I've spent so much time obsessing over my weight, I don't know what to do now. And I'm wondering when I need to stop doing this kind of work."

When we wonder, *When am I done?* we need to stop and ask a different question: *How can I make my journey more pleasurable?* This is life, and life is a process. Taking care of our physical and emotional health and wellness never ends. We're not here to find the finish line—we're here to enjoy the journey.

When we let go of limiting beliefs and emotions, life becomes even more amazing than we could have ever imagined. Even then, however, we never get to that moment when we don't have a single doubt or insecurity. The difference is that when we hear those voices, they no longer control us. We realize that emotions like joy, happiness, and gratitude are always within our reach.

Caring for the body and learning to love it even more continues to be a daily practice long after we've lost weight. Just as we don't shower once and say, "Well, that's it! I'm so clean now, I never need to shower again," we're never done with this process. While we're becoming our best selves and living our best lives, we can't help but pick up more dirt along the way. It's part of the human experience.

Using tapping on a regular basis, we're able to stay grounded in the body. When we hear those voices in our heads saying, "You're not good enough" or "You're not pretty enough" or "You can't do this," we can remind ourselves that these voices are just little mounds of dirt that we need to clear away; they're not who we are. When we hear them, we don't need to panic. Instead, we can regularly use tapping to clear them, the same way we shower regularly.

Through tapping, we also stay tuned in to what we need in body, mind, and soul. We can release the need to "fix" ourselves and "finish" the journey, and be present with what is, right now. We then see more clearly how food and movement affect us; we sense the body's need for more sleep or more fulfillment at work or more open communication in our relationships. The more we learn about how this amazing body of ours works, the more fascinating it is and the easier it is to live in a way that supports the body, so the body can support us in turn.

We find that when we allow ourselves to be present in our own lives, the journey feels much bigger and more rewarding than those so-called "after" pictures could ever be. We transform from the inside out, always loving ourselves and our bodies more and more. While the weight loss and renewed health and vitality feel great, we soon realize that shedding the weight was just a side effect of our commitment to express greater love toward ourselves.

In order to step fully into this larger journey, however, we must first let go of the resistance many of us experience, whether consciously or unconsciously. That's what we'll explore in this chapter.

## What Should I Do When I Fall Off the Wagon?

One of the most common questions I hear is, "What should I do when I fall off the wagon?" Unless you're a character from *Little House on the Prairie*, chances are you have rarely, if ever, been on a wagon. And since you're reading this book, I'll assume you're not on one now.

*There is no wagon.* This is your life. Just as when we search for a finish line that doesn't exist, when we worry about falling off some imaginary wagon or believe we've already fallen, we rob ourselves of the power of being present in the moment. If we gain some weight or eat in a manner that isn't ideal, instead of shaming ourselves we can simply choose something better next time: a more loving thought and action.

When you get caught up in the mentality of having fallen off an imaginary wagon, begin by getting clear on what emotions come up: anger, frustration, sadness? Allow those feelings to be your tapping targets. Then tap on your beliefs around the wagon itself. This tapping script may help you to begin integrating this new way of thinking.

**Karate Chop:** Even though I feel like I fell off the wagon, I accept myself. (*Repeat three times.*)

**Eyebrow:** I fell off the wagon.

**Side of Eye:** I was doing so well.

**Under Eye:** I was so motivated . . .

**Under Nose:** And then I messed up.

**Chin:** I made a mistake . . .

**Collarbone:** And I fell off the wagon.

**Under Arm:** I was doing perfectly . . .

**Top of Head:** Then I messed it all up.

**Eyebrow:** There is no wagon.

**Side of Eye:** This is my life.

**Under Eye:** I have this moment . . .

**Under Nose:** To choose a more loving thought and action.

**Chin:** Perfection is a myth.

## Hello, Old Pattern

I still fall into old patterns myself, but when I notice myself going into one I literally say, "Oh, hello, old pattern. I don't have time for you." Then I choose a different pattern. I don't need to panic, call myself a failure, or throw my hands up in the air because I'm "hopeless." Instead, I feel proud and excited every time I catch myself falling into it, that sneaky little bugger! Then I get curious. *Do I have more tapping to do or have I just slid into the familiar because I haven't practiced a newer and healthier pattern enough?*

**Collarbone:** I find peace in this moment.

**Under Arm:** I'm exactly where I'm meant to be.

**Top of Head:** I take action now to love and care for my body.

*Take a deep breath and check in with how you feel. If certain emotions, like frustration or anger, come up, be more specific with your tapping and target those until you experience relief.*

## The Weight of Perfection

Carolyn's love affair with dance began in college. Dancing felt like who she was, so when she wasn't sleeping, she was sure to be dancing. One day as she was leaving dance class, her teacher, who was also a famous modern dance choreographer, stopped her. Looking at Carolyn with disapproval that bordered on disgust, she told Carolyn that she'd never make it as a dancer with "that body." Carolyn either needed to stop eating or abandon the dream of a professional career in dance, she said. Stunned and heartbroken, Carolyn soon transferred to a major in acting, which still allowed her to dance but less often.

Now a mother of two, Carolyn has long been dreaming of teaching yoga but has felt too ashamed of her body to try. Since college, not being perfectly skinny has meant that she can't use or show her body in that way. After expressing her fears to the women in

*. . . if you have good thoughts, they will shine out of your face like sunbeams and you will always look lovely.*

—ROALD DAHL

my class, Carolyn was quickly overwhelmed by their support. Over and over again, women wrote in that they wished they could learn yoga from someone who wasn't perfect, but real. What she had long seen as her biggest flaw—not being "perfectly skinny"—was no longer an obstacle to sharing her talents.

As women, we are taught that having high standards is good and that striving for perfection makes us more valuable. The truth, though, is that the pressure to be the perfect amount of everything is driving us all crazy. From one day to the next, we're supposed to be thin but not too skinny; beautiful but not too sexy; strong but also feminine; caring but not too emotional; independent but not cold; confident but not self-absorbed; nurturing but not self-sacrificing. When we try to apply these standards to having the perfect weight loss journey, body, nutrition, exercise schedule, or even the perfect tapping experience, we find that "perfect" is never perfect enough.

Then we give up on ourselves because we think, *What's the point of trying so hard if I can't ever be good enough? If I can't be perfectly beautiful, I might as well wear baggy pants and an oversized sweatshirt again. There's no point in making my hair look nice,* we tell ourselves, *when my thighs look like this. I can't spend time on myself or my self-care because I'm too big,* we say. *I can't realize my dreams, speak my mind, pursue my ideas, or share what I know until I lose the weight.*

The pressure to be perfect and look perfect is never ending and all consuming. Our desperation for perfection makes us feel hopeless and out of control. Then we go from eating one chocolate to eating the entire bag because we believe we've already ruined this attempt at the perfect diet. The idea that there is a perfect diet, weight, and "after–weight loss" life where we have perfect thighs, butts, stomachs—and careers, homes, and relationships—is a belief that prevents us from feeling happy now.

We are women. We are emotional human beings, and sometimes we are more graceful than at other times. That's okay. That's how we're supposed to be. We don't need to be or look perfect, but we do need to allow ourselves to be in the present moment and to love ourselves and feel good in our bodies, regardless of our weight, as often as possible.

The key to success in this journey is realizing that we *are* good enough exactly the way we are right now. We don't need to live up to anything or meet anyone's expectations to be worthy. We don't need to live a life other than our own or try to make our life seem more like our friends' Facebook lives. We need to make peace with ourselves and believe that we really are good enough as we are. That's why we use tapping and continue this process, even after we lose the weight.

## Reconnecting Heart, Mind, and Body

The solution to this epidemic of perfection is to get out of our heads and into our bodies. When we connect with ourselves at a core level, we begin to value what we think more than what other people think.

What I love about tapping is how quickly and powerfully it can connect us to our bodies. When we feel that connection, we don't need to think about how to be perfect. Instead we *feel* what it really means to be ourselves. We take care of our bodies, not to please someone else or to live up to an ideal but because we believe in our own worth. *That* is when we can create sustainable change.

Gail shared her thoughts on perfection after realizing that for years she had been trying to be perfect to gain other people's approval. "I get it now—the praise, acknowledgment, love, and appreciation will just never be enough to make me happy as long as it comes only from an external source. I have been trying to be perfect to please others and to feel good about myself, yet I can never get what I need from others . . .

So, I try harder to be even more perfect so that maybe then I'll get the response I crave and *then* I'll feel good about myself. But that's just not going to happen while I am looking outside of myself for the emotions I crave to feel inside."

It's as true for Gail as it is for all of us: without self-acceptance and self-love, the approval and love we get from others will never be enough.

When we fully embrace this journey, we stop seeking perfection. Instead, we seek progress. We don't seek an answer; we seek relief. That's how we take steps forward and enjoy the journey. Until we can move forward in this way, we get stuck trying to figure out the answer instead of discovering it as we go, one step at a time.

## The Perfect Body

While at a family reunion one day, I commented to my aunt Penny that even though some of my cousins are blonde, what all the Ortners have in common are our signature full lips. "Oh yeah, it's unfortunate," she replied. I looked at her, confused. "Penny, women are injecting their lips to have fuller lips!" Shaking her head, she said, "Oh no, when I was growing up, it was the style to have really thin, delicate lips."

When it comes to the latest reasons to hate our bodies, it can be hard to keep up! We dislike body parts because they don't meet trends that are constantly changing. As we face record high rates of obesity, the standard for female beauty is thin, muscular women with boyish figures. The parts that distinguish us as women—hips, thighs, and rounder bellies—are what we often call "problem areas." But then, let's not forget, thanks to celebrities like Jennifer

> Being thought of as a beautiful woman has spared me nothing in life. No heartache, no trouble. Love has been difficult. Beauty is essentially meaningless and it is always transitory.
>
> —HALLE BERRY

Lopez and Beyoncé, having a rounder butt is now seen as fashionable. Again, it's hard to keep up!

Can we take a moment to contemplate how ridiculous this is? We shame the body we have for not being perfect but then don't hesitate to change our definition of "perfect" as soon as trends change. My friend Dr. Erin Shannon, who uses tapping with her professional athlete clients, shared that many top athletes suffer deeply from this "perfect" body ideal. She has found that athletes have some of the lowest body confidence she's seen because they feel that their worth is dependent on how their bodies look. As a result, they're constantly pointing out their bodies' so-called flaws.

The "perfect" body is a myth. Some of the women we are striving so hard to look like are just as tortured about having a "perfect" body as we are when we feel desperate to lose the weight. Without body confidence, none of us—including women we idolize for their "perfect" bodies—can feel good in our own skin.

Losing weight doesn't mean that negative self-talk and body shaming end or body confidence appears. While weight loss can improve

## When Am I My Ideal Weight?

People ask me this question often, but the answer is never up to me or to anyone other than you. The only way I can answer that question is by offering these ideas: You are your ideal weight when you don't turn to food as your only source of pleasure and relief. You are your ideal weight when you move your body as a way to show gratitude for all it does for you. You are your ideal weight when you begin to see your own beauty in the moment.

Regardless of your weight, you *are* ideal. You just have to be willing to recognize that.

health and well-being, even change how we feel in the body we currently have, it is never about becoming "perfect." Loving the body we're in can only happen from the inside out.

## Chasing "The Land of After"

Although I've already touched on how dangerous it is for us to chase the magical "land of after," it's such a common block for women that I want to take a moment to explore it in greater detail.

Many women I've worked with are tricked into believing in a magical land of "after weight loss," where everything will fall into place and be perfect. They secretly envision their careers becoming perfectly fulfilling, their relationships improving, and themselves being perfectly loved and adored by all.

Losing weight because we think that doing so will make everything in life perfect is only a lie we've been chasing. It's also a lie that robs us of the experience of living life in the present moment. It's the reason we don't allow ourselves to be happy and the reason we don't go for what we want and need.

Losing the weight will not improve our relationships. It will not improve our careers. We really need to wrap our heads around the fact that this is a lie we've been telling ourselves.

What's going to make these changes in our lives is the way we begin to feel about ourselves. Does that mean that you shouldn't lose some weight and enjoy the health and vibrancy weight loss provides? Absolutely not. You deserve to experience how strong and energetic your physical body can feel, but when you have this idea that weight loss will deliver that utopian moment, you create stress that can interfere with your journey. If you're always waiting for the perfect moment, you can never enjoy the progress you've made because that progress never feels good enough.

When we embrace what is true and real in the present moment, we can feel grounded. Finally we can enjoy our lives! One of my students wrote about the freedom she had begun to experience by releasing the need for perfection: "I used to postpone things until I was in the perfect shape, or could do something in a perfect way, or have perfect acknowledgment from others," she shared. "After tapping and working with this weight loss process, I now do things first. The result is that every day I feel better and better."

Another student wrote, "I have discovered that it was precisely my wish to be the 'perfect mom' and 'perfect wife' that kept me from trying or even starting to just *be me*. Tapping helped me get over the idea that I needed to be perfect."

When we release the need for perfection, we can also develop and grow in a conscious, gentle, and natural way.

## Self-Improvement: Proceed with Caution

Throughout this book we've discussed the power of awareness. As conscious and caring women, many of us are actively seeking ways to develop ourselves both internally and externally. While this intention is a positive one, we also need to be aware that it can work against us.

> To make mistakes is human;
> to stumble is commonplace;
> to be able to laugh at
> yourself is maturity.
>
> —WILLIAM ARTHUR WARD

As we saw at the end of the last chapter, self-development is not self-care. Too often our emphasis on self-improvement goes one step further and turns into self-punishment. When we have the mentality that we are broken, we will always find something to fix. Because tapping is so powerful, it can be easy to fall into this way of thinking. We clear an issue only to find another and then think, *I've got a lot more work to do on myself*. In this way, we rob ourselves of the experience of feeling relief and relaxation for having cleared one issue because we're already focused on the next.

When we have amazing results with tapping, we can also fall into the trap of thinking that since tapping is so effective, we should never feel a negative emotion again. That's not how life (or tapping!) works.

Life would be boring if it were always the same—always calm and placid and upbeat. A beautiful song, like life, is made up of high and low notes. The contrast between the ups and downs is what makes us appreciate each one and truly feel alive. Tapping doesn't control the future or numb us from ever feeling a tough emotion; it helps us move through the melody and appreciate life's many different notes.

As you move forward in this journey using tapping to address your challenges, I hope you will always remember this: *You are not a problem that needs to be solved. Your focus should be on finding new and better ways to continue loving and accepting yourself.*

Yes, this journey can get serious, but no matter how bumpy the ride may feel at times, remember always that there is nothing wrong with you. You are growing, evolving, and learning new ways to love

## Beware of Idolizing

Katharine Hepburn, Marilyn Monroe, and Mother Teresa all had their share of stinky farts, some of which they probably blamed on the dog. We are all human. We all feel sadness and joy. At some level we are all afraid of rejection. We are all emotional human beings trying to do our best.

We look at other women and idolize them and their lives. We compare our lives with the lives they show to the public and feel "less than," not good enough.

If we are busy idolizing someone else's life and someone else's body, we don't have time and energy to cultivate a relationship with our own life and body.

Instead of idolizing or comparing yourself, get curious. What traits do they have that you would like to express? Jealousy is simply a longing to wake up to our own power. Celebrate other people's achievements, knowing that just like them, you can do great things.

yourself, your body, and your life. This process never needs to be "perfect" for it to transform how you feel and then how you look.

If we are going to embark on this voyage of self-discovery, we also need to remember that we won't survive without a sense of humor. The more pain we feel, the more we need to remember to laugh. Laughter is a great antidote to perfection because it gets us out of our heads and into our bodies. That's why I'd rather make light of cellulite than demonize it.

## So . . . What Are We Reaching For?

As we've seen, the point of this journey isn't to look like a digitally edited photo of a model or to give up on ourselves and surrender to all the health challenges that come with being overweight. The point is to figure out how to take care of *us*. We are all at our most powerful when we are our healthiest. To be our healthiest, we need to allow ourselves to experience true emotional freedom.

## The Freedom to Feel

If there is one thing I hope you get from this book, it's the ability to release your fear of feeling. As women, we are so often told that we are "too emotional." We hide our feelings because we don't want to be called "crazy" or "too sensitive." Yet our ability to feel deeply is our greatest gift. It makes us compassionate and intuitive. It enables us to nurture ourselves and those we love. It makes us the amazing women we are.

Our goal isn't to be happy all the time and then shame ourselves whenever we don't look and feel like a ray of sunshine. The goal is to realize that we don't have to be victims of circumstance and then do what we need to do to feel better more often.

Through tapping, we can embrace our many different emotions and have the freedom to feel enthusiastic, even when we meet disappointment. That's what happens when we're no longer afraid to experience a full range of emotions. Because we know we can handle disappointment, we simply learn from it and try a different approach next time. For the same reason, we can feel happy and safe even while knowing that the future is uncertain, as it always will be.

The more we accept ourselves and our emotions, the less drama we tend to create during challenging moments. Instead of punishing ourselves or our loved ones, we can feel what we feel, tap, take action (if needed), and then move on.

> Those who don't know how to weep with their whole heart don't know how to laugh either.
>
> —GOLDA MEIR

Confidence doesn't come from thinking we'll never again be thrown overboard by rough waters, but from knowing that we *will* get thrown over—and that we will continue to grow and thrive, using tapping to support us in navigating the storms. The more we can find peace with that fact, the more we can trust the process and enjoy ourselves through the calm and stormy seasons of our lives. We can even appreciate that storms help us see how powerful and capable we really are.

## Hello, Me, It's Nice to Meet You

When we've spent many years denying our own worth and stuffing down emotions, taking time to focus on ourselves can feel unnatural. As one student wrote, "Sometimes I feel that I've released so much that I have to meet my present self all over again because with the layers of the onion being stripped away goes most of my story. I've realized that I am not my anxiety or depression, and with them being released I'm not at all sure who I am. It's like living with a stranger."

As we move forward on this journey, we need to continue spending time learning what we love and what lights us up. We need to

## Exiting Your Comfort Zone

Trying something new (a new workout class, a new project, even kale!) is scary because we are conditioned to fear the unknown.

One of my favorite sayings from yoga is "Find the ease in the pose." It can feel uncomfortable to move your body in new ways and stretch your perceived limits, but once you find the ease in the pose, the pose becomes easier.

If we simply seek what's safe and comfortable, we end up on the couch eating out of a bag. To truly live, you need to expand beyond your comfort zone. There's no need to judge yourself for feeling a bit uncomfortable; it's a part of growing. Tapping can help you find ease in this new zone.

spend time figuring out what we believe in. As we use tapping to pull out the weeds, we must spend time planting new seeds. Throughout this book I have shared positive tapping phrases. They're powerful in their own right. These are the vitamins that keep you strong. Take them daily.

## Celebrate Every Small Step

Many of us have fallen into a pattern of waiting for "results" before we allow ourselves to celebrate, but a crucial part of enjoying the journey is noticing and celebrating our progress. We can't hold off celebrating until we've lost our first 20 or 50 pounds; we have to celebrate each and every small victory along the way.

Donna experienced this when she had her first breakthrough during my class. One day while working at home, she felt munchy and spotted a bag of chocolate candies in the fridge that her teenage son had left behind. She was surprised her son had done that because Donna was notorious in the family for having little self-control around chocolate. But this time after eating a few pieces, she realized that the candy didn't taste good to her. Then she realized that she wasn't actually hungry at all. Without any struggle or regret, she returned the bag of candy to the fridge, feeling no desire to eat more. It wasn't until later that the magnitude of that moment hit her. As she said, "This would *never* have happened before."

For Donna, this was a huge moment and she was proud of herself. The more we celebrate the small shifts, the more shifts we feel comfortable making and the more we enjoy the process. Physical changes may take time, but as the old saying goes, "Time flies when you're having fun."

# Embracing the Journey Forward

**Eyebrow:** I'm so proud of myself.

**Side of Eye:** I've come so far.

**Under Eye:** I honor where I am . . .

**Under Nose:** And I'm ready for the next step.

**Chin:** I embrace my life now.

**Collarbone:** I enjoy this journey.

**Under Arm:** I am exactly where I am meant to be.

**Top of Head:** It feels so good to feel good.

**Eyebrow:** I appreciate my body with loving words.

**Side of Eye:** When I notice an unkind voice . . .

**Under Eye:** I find power in the present moment . . .

**Under Nose:** And choose to be kind.

**Chin:** I promise to stand by the person in the mirror . . .

**Collarbone:** Even when she makes a mistake.

**Under Arm:** Disapproving of myself hasn't been working.

**Top of Head:** I now choose to love and approve of myself.

**Eyebrow:** As there is movement in my body . . .

**Side of Eye:** There is movement in my life.

**Under Eye:** I experience creativity and gratitude through movement.

**Under Nose:** I fall deeper in love with movement.

**Chin:** I begin to notice what foods are best for my body.

**Collarbone:** There is no place to arrive to.

**Under Arm:** I'm constantly learning what my body needs.

**Top of Head:** I create a loving relationship with my body and food.

**Eyebrow:** I make pleasure a priority.

**Side of Eye:** I find easy ways to add more pleasure to my life.

**Under Eye:** I give myself moments to simply relax.

**Under Nose:** As I learn to say no to others . . .

**Chin:** I say yes to myself.

**Collarbone:** As I begin to value my time . . .

**Under Arm:** Others begin to value my time.

**Top of Head:** It's safe to put my well-being first.

**Eyebrow:** It's safe for me to shine.

**Side of Eye:** I'm pulled forward toward my dreams.

**Under Eye:** I have the courage and faith I need.

**Under Nose:** I let go of what other people think . . .

**Chin:** And honor what I think.

**Collarbone:** This journey is about me . . .

**Under Arm:** And as I allow myself to shine . . .

**Top of Head:** I inspire others to do the same.

**Eyebrow:** I release the need to find every answer.

**Side of Eye:** I release the need to solve every problem.

**Under Eye:** I can be happy now, exactly where I am.

**Under Nose:** It's never been about the weight.

**Chin:** The weight was just trying to get my attention . . .

**Collarbone:** To wake me up to my potential.

**Under Arm:** I experience my power by caring for my body.

**Top of Head:** I love, accept, and thank my incredible body for leading me here.

# Conclusion

During my class as women share their experiences with one another, I often hear them say, "I thought it was just me." They're amazed by how much they have in common and how many similar experiences they've had with food, weight, exercise, and much more.

Because we have felt so much pressure to be perfect, we often isolate ourselves from other women who could support us. That holds us back on our journey because, as we've seen, what we need is not more struggle but more love and support. When we're on this journey toward weight loss and body confidence, we need to know that no matter what we are going through, there are many other women who feel what we're feeling.

As I see over and over again in groups of thousands of online students, when we're willing to be honest and open with one another, we realize that we aren't so different. The more open we can be about how we really feel, the less shame we have. I'm not talking about sitting around in a circle singing "Kumbaya," or the other extreme of sitting around complaining to each other. I'm talking about allowing ourselves to be real and compassionate toward one another.

As one student shared, "This group provides something I have been looking for for 54 years—acceptance. It is so powerful, and it helps me accept and love myself. It is safe to ask for help, and no one has told me to try harder or suggested that what I bring to the table is not enough." Having a skewed relationship with food and body image is a lot more common than each of us thinks. The good news is that with tapping, we have a tool to address it.

When we're able to accept ourselves and our feelings, we can open up about our struggles and seek out like-minded community and support. Instead of standing back, let's come together and wholeheartedly offer each other encouragement.

> Growing into your future . . . requires a dedication to caring for yourself as if you were rare and precious, which you are.
>
> —VICTORIA MORAN

Weeks after my online class ends, women continue to post on Facebook and cheer each other on. This kind of support is incredibly powerful and often has ripple effects throughout their lives. They often find themselves meeting new people outside the group as well and receiving new support. Whether or not you're part of an established group or network that can support you in this journey, I encourage you to stay open to the possibility of receiving support from others as well. It often happens in ways and at times you don't expect.

While running a 5k with my mom one day, I had a great reminder about the power of community support. As I was approaching the finish line, I was blown away by the excitement and enthusiasm of the crowd cheering all of us runners on. It was an incredible feeling. I was tired, but hearing the cheers gave me the extra fuel I needed to finish.

Once I was done running, I took a spot on the sidelines to cheer other runners on for a moment and then doubled back on the race route to cross the finish line a second time with my mom. As we crossed, the crowd's cheers were just as strong and just as loud as they had been the first time. I didn't know most of the people in the crowd, but I felt like I did. Their support had transformed a good race into a wonderful and inspiring experience. It was such a simple but profound reminder about the power of community. We all need support. I, for one, am cheering you on!

# I Thought This Was a Weight Loss Book?

My favorite comment of all time came from a student in my online course who wrote, "Thank you, Jessica, for tricking us with the title of this course. What I think you were really creating was a movement for empowering women to transform our lives, get our energies flowing, strut our stuff, make the world a better place, and fall in love with life . . . with the helpful side effects of losing weight and living longer, happier, healthier lives! And I am so grateful!!"

My eyes filled with tears when I first read this because it captures so perfectly why I do the work I do. We're women. We can't compartmentalize our lives. So often, when we want nothing more than to lose weight, what we actually need is to stop trying to lose weight and simply start living.

The most powerful way I know for you to lose weight and feel great in your body is to use tapping to clear your limiting emotions and beliefs so you can start listening to your inner voice. It's time for you to start caring about what you think, so yes, go ahead and try that tango class, ask for a raise, and say no to people who drain you. Whatever your heart and body are telling you, it's time to listen. To experience all the incredible benefits of this process, you must take the time to do the tapping. This process doesn't work if you don't make tapping a priority in your life. Even just ten minutes in the morning can be enough to transform your entire day.

This journey is not about food and it's not about exercise. While the journey can and should include positive and empowering changes in both of those areas (and many others), those changes need to happen as part of a larger and more important process if they're going to lead to long-term body confidence and weight loss.

We know we're fully immersed in the journey when instead of dreading movement, we exercise because it feels so good to do it. When instead of counting calories or shaming ourselves for eating something "bad," we find we're eating more fresh and wholesome food because it's delicious and it nourishes us in body and soul. When instead of hiding in the shadows, we take care of ourselves and delight in the pleasure that surrounds us. We know we're succeeding in moving forward in our journey when we allow ourselves to look and feel beautiful and share our many gifts with a world that needs nothing more than for us to shine brighter and brighter every single day.

From this place we can be loving and open, ready and able to adapt to change. From here, we don't need things to always stay the same or feel easy. We know our bodies will change as the years pass just as we know that our hearts will expand and our gifts will deepen. But from this new home inside ourselves, we no longer fear these changes. Because we have come to deeply love and accept ourselves, we can savor the ride and feel grateful for the bumps we encounter, knowing that they're here to remind us of what we must not forget: that life is happening right now, and that we can and must delight in it and love ourselves just as we are now.

It's not about the weight; it's never been about the weight. This is about your life, your power, and the courage to shine.

# Resources

I'd like to share some books and resources I have enjoyed while on my own journey to weight loss and body confidence. Many of these I have referenced within the book.

*The Art of Extreme Self-Care: Transform Your Life One Month at a Time,* by Cheryl Richardson

*The Biology of Belief: Unleashing the Power of Consciousness, Matter, and Miracles,* by Bruce H. Lipton, Ph.D.

*The Blood Sugar Solution: The UltraHealthy Program for Losing Weight, Preventing Disease, and Feeling Great Now!,* by Mark Hyman, M.D.

*The First 30 Days: Your Guide to Making Any Change Easier,* by Ariane de Bonvoisin

*The Gabriel Method: The Revolutionary Diet-Free Way to Totally Transform Your Body,* by Jon Gabriel

*In Defense of Food: An Eater's Manifesto,* by Michael Pollan

*Mind Over Medicine: Scientific Proof that You Can Heal Yourself,* by Lissa Rankin, M.D.

*Mindless Eating: Why We Eat More Than We Think,* by Brian Wansink, Ph.D.

*Remembering Wholeness: A Personal Handbook for Thriving in the 21st Century,* by Carol Tuttle

*Salt Sugar Fat: How the Food Giants Hooked Us,* by Michael Moss

*The Slow Down Diet: Eating for Pleasure, Energy, and Weight Loss,* by Marc David

*The Tapping Solution: A Revolutionary System for Stress-Free Living,* by Nick Ortner

*Women, Food, and God: An Unexpected Path to Almost Everything,* by Geneen Roth

*Women's Bodies, Women's Wisdom: Creating Physical and Emotional Health and Healing,* by Christiane Northrup, M.D.

*You Can Heal Your Life,* by Louise L. Hay

For a full list, direct links, and bonus material you can go to www.TheTappingSolution.com/resources

# Index

# Acknowledgments

"Thank you" are two little words that can never express the depth of my gratitude for the countless people who have helped this book come to life and supported me throughout this journey.

Thank you to my brothers, best friends, and business partners, Nick and Alex. You tease me enough to keep me grounded while always standing by me and blowing wind in my sails. Nick, I am where I am today because of your love, unshakable faith, and crazy ideas. You never let anything distract you from your sincere passion to make the world a better place. You inspire me every day. Alex, none of this would have been possible without your brilliant mind and loving heart. You breathe life into ideas that are changing lives, all while doing movie impressions that leave me laughing until I'm wiping tears from my face. I look up to both of you not because you're my big brothers but because you're incredible human beings.

Mom and Dad, thank you for supporting me when I chose the road less traveled. I'm grateful to be your daughter. I love you. Brenna, having a sister-in-law who's been your best friend since seventh grade is very convenient when it comes to fact-checking your own book! I'm grateful for every moment of our friendship. Karen, I will always cherish the time we spent together while working on this book. Thank you for opening your beautiful home to me. To my nephews, Malakai and Lucas, and my niece, Olivia, people may doubt that a four-year-old, two-year-old, and eight-month-old could help me write a book, but you helped me more than I can express. Your laughter and love always lifted my spirits whenever I had doubts. To Deirdre Mammano and Sarah Dade, some people are born with sisters and others find them on their path through life. I'm grateful I found you. To the rest of my incredible family and friends, this has been possible because of you.

There are so many people who have helped bring this book to life. Reid Tracy, I'll never forget that phone call when you told me I had to write this book. I was so scared, but your faith gave me wings. I am forever grateful. Patty Gift, you are an incredible friend and brilliant editor. Thank you for believing in my vision. To Wyndham Wood, the stars aligned when I met you. Thank you for your love and support. To Louise Hay, Dr. Christiane Northrup, Cheryl Richardson, Dr. Lissa Rankin, Ariane de Bonvoisin, Laura Gray, Autumn Millhouse, Mary Ayers, Michelle Polizzi, Ellie Jacque-Capon, Erin Stutland—deep bow in gratitude! Thank you to Nick Polizzi, the director and editor of *The Tapping Solution*. I will never forget unpacking all the film equipment in my brother's tiny one-bedroom apartment and realizing what an enormous leap of faith we were all taking. I'm grateful we leapt together.

Thank you to everyone at The Tapping Solution. None of this would be possible without this incredible team. Thank you to the countless tapping and personal development experts who have let me interview them. Everything I know is because I have stood on the shoulders of giants. My heart is filled with gratitude.

# ABOUT THE AUTHOR

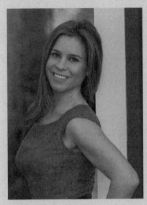

**Jessica Ortner** is a producer of *The Tapping Solution,* the breakthrough documentary film on EFT/meridian tapping (www.TheTappingSolution. com). She has led more than 3,000 women through her revolutionary Weight Loss and Body Confidence online programme, and she is also the host of The Tapping World Summit, an annual online event that has attracted more than 500,000 attendees from around the world. She has been interviewing experts in the personal development field since 2007, having conducted more than 200 broadcast interviews to date. Follow Jessica on Twitter @JessicaOrtner and on Facebook at www.facebook. com/followingJessicaOrtner.

www.jessica-ortner.com

We hope you enjoyed this Hay House book. If you'd like to receive our online catalog featuring additional information on Hay House books and products, or if you'd like to find out more about the Hay Foundation, please contact:

Hay House UK, Ltd.,
Astley House, 33 Notting Hill Gate, London W11 3JQ
*Phone:* 0-20-3675-2450 • *Fax:* 0-20-3675-2451
www.hayhouse.co.uk • www.hayfoundation.org

**Published and distributed in the United States by:**
Hay House, Inc., P.O. Box 5100, Carlsbad, CA 92018-5100
*Phone:* (760) 431-7695 or (800) 654-5126
*Fax:* (760) 431-6948 or (800) 650-5115
www.hayhouse.com®

**Published and distributed in Australia by:** Hay House Australia Pty. Ltd.,
18/36 Ralph St., Alexandria NSW 2015 • *Phone:* 612-9669-4299 • *Fax:* 612-9669-4144 •
www.hayhouse.com.au

**Published and distributed in the Republic of South Africa by:** Hay House SA (Pty), Ltd.,
P.O. Box 990, Witkoppen 2068 • *Phone/Fax:* 27-11-467-8904 • www.hayhouse.co.za

**Published in India by:** Hay House Publishers India, Muskaan Complex, Plot No. 3, B-2,
Vasant Kunj, New Delhi 110 070 • *Phone:* 91-11-4176-1620 • *Fax:* 91-11-4176-1630 •
www.hayhouse.co.in

**Distributed in Canada by:** Raincoast Books, 2440 Viking Way, Richmond, B.C. V6V 1N2
*Phone:* 1-800-663-5714 • *Fax:* 1-800-565-3770 • www.raincoast.com

TAKE YOUR SOUL ON A VACATION

Visit www.HealYourLife.com® to regroup, recharge, and reconnect with your own magnificence.
Featuring blogs, mind-body-spirit news, and life-changing wisdom from Louise Hay and friends.

Visit www.HealYourLife.com today!

**Keep up the joyous momentum with these free bonuses by visiting me at**

**www.TheTappingSolution.com/ReadyToShine**

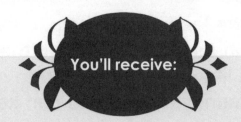

You'll receive:

Extended interviews with experts featured in the book

Tapping meditation audio "Feeling Safe to Shine"

Free *Tapping In The Morning and Evening for Stress Relief* CD

"How to Tap" wallet card

Helpful handouts

Printable PDF of each tapping meditation featured in the book!

**Ready to join the program and supportive community today?**

**The Tapping Solution "Weight Loss & Body Confidence 7-Week Program"**
**Use coupon code *"ready2shine"* to save an extra 10%!**

www.TheTappingSolution.com/confidence